Care That Works

Care That Works

A Relationship Approach
to Persons with Dementia

JITKA M. ZGOLA

The Johns Hopkins University Press
Baltimore and London

An earlier version of Chapter 10 was published as "Alzheimer's Disease and the Home: Issues in Environmental Design," *American Journal of Alzheimer's Disease and Related Disorders and Research* (May–June 1990). An earlier version of the section on the Tea Group in Chapter 12 first appeared as "The Tea Group: A Special Program for the 'Difficult' Residents in Long-Term Care," *Physical and Occupational Therapy in Geriatrics* 10, no. 3 (1992): 1–16. An earlier version of Chapter 13 was presented at the Ninth National Conference on Gerontological Nursing in Toronto, June 1991.

The Johns Hopkins University Press
2715 North Charles Street
Baltimore, Maryland 21218-4363
www.press.jhu.edu

Library of Congress Cataloging-in-Publication Data will be found at the end of this book.
A catalog record for this book is available from the British Library.

ISBN 0-8018-6025-3
ISBN 0-8018-6026-1 (pbk.)

Contents

Preface and Acknowledgments

A principal constituent of a positive relationship is respect. This does not necessarily mean admiration or favor; it simply means unconditional regard for the person as she is. Regard grows from understanding. Alzheimer's disease can make it very difficult for the caregiver to understand the affected person. It distorts that individual's behavior, obscures her intentions and motivations, and clouds her history. The first part of this book, therefore, deals with getting to know the effects of the illness that the person is living with. It begins by defining, in functional terms, dementia and other terms commonly used in association with the illness. It outlines the most common effects of dementing illness on behavior and function. This book does not describe dementing illness from the biomedical and clinical perspective; it deals exclusively with psychosocial management from an intra- and interpersonal perspective.

Because ongoing information gathering is an essential part of effective care, part of the book is dedicated to the process of observation, gathering historical information, and functional evaluation that would be done as part of continuing care. It describes ways of assessing the person's current cognitive and functional abilities, and follows with approaches to gathering history about the person and her life and times. All this information is then brought together to help the caregiver prevent and contain challenging behaviors.

Interventions are discussed from three general perspectives: interpersonal relationships, environments, and activities. Interpersonal relationships are built through effective communication and problem-solving processes. The discussion of environment goes beyond bricks-and-mortar issues; it includes social as well as cultural elements. The social environment refers to the interpersonal contacts that affect the person. The cultural environment refers to shared values, traditions, history, routines, and alliances that characterize a group of people who live and work together. The section on activities invites caregivers to examine some basic concepts regarding occupation, its nature and purpose, in the context of dementing illness. It examines activity programming in the home and in the residential setting.

This is not a technical treatise on Alzheimer's disease. It is a collection of ideas and experiences gathered over years of trying to make sense of a situation where the principal feature seems to be that things do not make sense and the principal objective is simply to make things work to the benefit of everyone concerned.

The reader who starts at page 1 and continues through to the end will find many instances of repetition. This is because the boundaries between issues treated in each chapter are not precise and elements from one affect another. Also, there is an advantage to looking at any issue from more than one angle. Therefore, any one issue treated in this book is worked into several different frames of reference. This repetition of concepts and information is also a conscious compromise of elegance to accommodate professionals and family caregivers, whose busy lives seldom permit cover-to-cover reading. It is done so that each chapter can more or less stand alone in the treatment of a particular topic.

This book is directed to both family and professional care providers. Some chapters deal with the home situation specifically, while others pertain more to the professional care setting. Nonetheless, the principles discussed can be applied to either situation. It was conceived this way with the intention of attracting family caregivers to read material geared to professional care providers and professionals to read material aimed at family caregivers. Optimal care depends on families and professional caregivers communicating well with one another and supporting each other in their common objective, which is meeting the needs of the cognitively impaired person. If they are to communicate well, they must operate with the same concepts and use a common vocabulary. One step toward developing such coherence is to read the same material.

Finally, this book reflects on the fact that each encounter, in the continuing effort to help another person cope with the challenges of dementing illness, has the potential to teach us something. We might discover another dimension in the person for whom we are caring and might also find another dimension in ourselves that has appeared as a consequence of the caring situation. Many of these lessons will be wonderfully applicable to all our relationships. They are, no doubt, different for everyone. However, a starting list might be the following:

- Although you may be able to influence the behavior of another person, the only behavior you can really control is your own.
- Walk a mile in the other person's shoes, or at least try really hard to imagine what it might be like, before committing yourself to a judgment about another person's behavior.
- Always make it possible for the other person to save face.

- Treat yourself with as much tolerance, forgiveness, and understanding as you do the people you care for.
- It is a lot easier to know what needs to be done than to do it.

This book is a reflection of some fifteen years spent in the company of several hundred remarkable people, people who have been forced, by a terrible illness, to search for new ways of coping with life. Their efforts and those of their families, friends, neighbors, counselors, and helpers have provided the substance of this book. I extend thanks to them all for the lessons that came from their letting me share in the struggle, the fear, the anger, the joy, the laughter, and the living. If these lessons are expressed accurately and effectively, it is also due to the technical support of respected colleagues: Anne Carswell, Ph.D., associate professor and director, Rehabilitation Sciences, University of British Columbia, Vancouver; Guy Proulx, Ph.D., director of psychology, Baycrest Hospital, Toronto; and Barbara Collins, psychologist, Ottawa General Hospital, Ottawa.

Care That Works

1 | Relationships

The aim of effective care is to support a quality of life that respects the dignity, identity, and needs of both the person in care and the caregiver. This kind of care is possible only in the context of a trusting and mutually respectful relationship. In the presence of such a relationship, caring can be an enriching experience; in its absence, it becomes a custodial affair.

Although the merit of a trusting and mutually respectful relationship is not limited to the care of persons with Alzheimer's disease, it has a special place in dementia care. First, dementing illness renders the affected person not only physically but also emotionally dependent on the caregiver. The affected person relies, moment by moment, on his environment and the people in it for feedback about his security and sense of worth. Second, without memory, insight, and judgment, a cognitively impaired person cannot compensate for or accommodate to the inconsistencies, miscommunications, and oversights that are part of normal human interaction. It is up to the caregivers to ensure that the messages the person receives are consistently supportive and affirming, that they build and never threaten his sense of value, identity, security, and control.

Dementing illness also creates situations that would be intensely challenging to any relationship. Although the person with Alzheimer's disease and the caregiver share the same world, they often perceive it from different perspectives. The cognitively impaired person may appear to see, hear, and otherwise experience the same things that the caregiver does. He may seem physically capable of the same responses. Yet his experience and reactions are affected by a profound distortion of both incoming and outgoing information. It is a distortion that he cannot explain, account for, or compensate for and of which he is usually not even aware. Due to this lack of insight, the person cannot meet the caregiver halfway, work things out, compromise, or otherwise contribute to the effort of building or preserving the relationship. The entire responsibility, therefore, rests with the caregiver.

Such a responsibility may, at first glance, appear overwhelming and unfairly arduous. How can anyone be expected to bear such a burden? Once a caregiver accepts this responsibility and acquires the necessary skills, he gains mastery over the situation. That is the objective of this book: to give the caregiver the insight and information with which to build and maintain a positive relationship.

The term *relationship* is used to refer to an alliance in which the caregiver aims to safeguard and promote the affected person's ability to meet basic human needs. The needs identified in this book are security, control, affection, and inclusion.

- *Security* refers not only to safety in an objective sense but also to the subjective feeling of freedom from threat, both physical and emotional.
- *Control* means having a say about the way in which one's own effects, person, time, and space are handled.
- *Affection* refers not only to being loved but also to being perceived as a loving person.
- *Inclusion* means being part of a collective, having a cohort, belonging.

These needs must be addressed in every encounter, no matter what a person's apparent receptivity. Even if the person fails to respond in a recognizable fashion to things that are going on, we cannot assume that he does not appreciate the feelings that are being projected and that he has no feelings in response. Unless we are consistently attentive to these needs, we could be not only depriving the person of vital experience but also inadvertently causing harm.

A person with dementia, affected by memory loss, perceptual disturbances, etc., is easily prone to feelings of lost control, insecurity, and vulnerability. A natural reaction to such feelings is to fight for control, look out for danger, or flee and seek solace. In such circumstances, it is only natural to turn to a trusted partner, someone who will help preserve one's sense of control instead of removing it, provide support in the face of frightening events instead of contributing to them, and offer comfort and resolution. When a person with Alzheimer's disease can find such a partnership in his caregiver, problems do not necessarily evaporate, but they do become manageable. This is the aim of caring: to establish an alliance in which the cognitively impaired person and the caregiver are able to do whatever needs to be done in the course of daily living and, when problems occur, to manage them together. The ability to forge such an alliance comes out of a number of elements on the part of the caregiver:

- understanding the challenges that a person with Alzheimer's disease faces in each encounter;
- awareness of and regard for the person's personality, habits, and identity;
- awareness of and respect for the cognitively impaired person's needs;
- appreciation of and regard for the retained abilities that the person enlists in his effort to make sense of the world; and
- structuring each encounter with the person in a way that consistently compensates for deficits and promotes retained abilities.

Once this relationship is in place, it can carry the cognitively impaired person and the caregiver through some very rough times. In the security of this alliance, the person whose world is unpredictable and often threatening finds the strength to deal with situations that would otherwise provoke fear, resentment, or defensiveness. One need only feel the pressure of the cognitively impaired person's hand as he is led into the testing room or other frightening situation to appreciate the intensity of this trust and the extent of his vulnerability.

If the relationship is sound, a caregiver can also risk saying and doing things that may frighten or upset the person. One gentleman expressed deep gratitude for the fact that his wife trusted him even though he had lost his temper with her and said some very hurtful things. "If there is anything good about this disease," he said, "it's that, because she doesn't remember what I say from one moment to another, she doesn't remember the bad things either. She does remember, though, that we are sweethearts, that I love her, and that I would never let anything bad happen to her."

The concept of "relationship" and what it means to a cognitively impaired person needs closer examination. The better we understand it, the more powerful a tool it will become in our effort to provide for an optimum quality of life for both the cognitively impaired person and those caring for him.

We still have much to learn. The following example illustrates the power of relationship and how far we really are from being able to understand and exploit it.

Mrs. F. was very limited in her abilities. She initiated few activities and did little on request. Feeding her a meal took well over an hour. Her intake at each meal was so poor that it needed to be supplemented with frequent snacks. Her caregivers, all of whom felt that they had a good, respectful, and trusting relationship with her, spent much time and effort coaxing, reminding, and simply waiting for her to open her mouth for each spoonful. Even when given her favorite foods, she appeared simply to have forgotten how to eat. Everyone believed that this was due to her advanced dementia and that patience was the only resource available to them. One day, as Mrs. F. was having lunch, macaroni and cheese, the two-year-old boy whom her caregiver was babysitting came around, reached into her bowl, picked up a piece of macaroni in his fingers, and fed it to her. Mrs. F. ate it out of his hand and eagerly waited for the next piece. She was alert to each morsel that he gave her. The only thing that limited the speed of her eating was the dexterity of the little boy's fingers.

What did this little boy awaken in Mrs. F. that her other caregivers could not reach, despite their well-intentioned and thoughtful efforts? What we see in a cognitively impaired person is not all there is. Our challenge is to learn how to reach what lies within.

This example also raises the question of who is a caregiver. The term *caregiver* is often used to describe the role of the one person who is most intimately and consistently involved with the day-to-day support of a cognitively impaired individual. In this example, we see that even a little boy can fulfill a significant caregiving role. In fact, everyone who comes into contact with such a person has some responsibility for making that encounter as supportive, meaningful, and comfortable as possible. For that, knowledge is essential.

Some time ago, we developed a program that involved a local museum bringing in artifacts that dated from the turn of the century (Zgola and Coulter 1988). The aim was to promote conversation, reminiscence, and self-esteem. The program, however, had an additional effect. The museum staff who brought us the artifacts learned how to interact with persons who had cognitive disabilities. On more than one occasion they reported that they had been able to spot cognitively impaired persons at the museum who were having difficulty understanding their tour, and were able to reorient and redirect them effectively because of insights they had gained in the program. They had become more effective caregivers in their jobs.

2	# Dementia:

Definition and Consequences

Understanding the Definition

The best way to understand another person's behavior is to try to put ourselves in that person's shoes. Insight into the effects of cognitive impairment will help us imagine how the world might appear to a person with Alzheimer's disease and how the illness might be affecting that person's reactions. If we look carefully and persistently enough, we can often see in a cognitively impaired person's behavior a rational effort to cope with circumstances that have ceased making sense to her.

Recognition of this rational aspect of behavior in a person with dementia is fundamental to the formation and maintenance of a caring relationship. It gives the cognitively impaired person credit for being a reasonable adult. If this person's behavior should become either problematic or simply difficult to understand, a caregiver who recognizes it as a rational response to circumstances will try to alter the circumstances rather than the behavior. The caregiver might even try to enlist the person's cooperation in dealing with the situation. This way, the caregiver's efforts are directed toward controlling the situation, not the person. When the caregiver exercises this control in partnership with the person, not in opposition to her, the alliance between them is strengthened, not weakened. This is done with the recognition that a cognitively impaired person is an adult with adult reactions. Just like any adult, she is likely to respond more favorably to guidance than to control.

This kind of sensitivity and responsiveness does not arise simply out of the caregiver's good will. It is possible only when the caregiver really understands the behavioral and functional effects of dementia. First we must take a close look at the classical definition.

The American Psychiatric Association's definition of dementia of the Alzheimer's type, in part, is:

A. The development of multiple cognitive deficits manifested by both:
    1) memory impairment (impaired ability to learn new information
        or to recall previously learned information)
    2) one (or more) of the following cognitive disturbances:
        a) aphasia (language disturbance)
        b) apraxia (impaired ability to carry out motor activities despite
            intact motor function)
        c) agnosia (failure to recognize or identify objects despite intact
            sensory function)
        d) disturbances in executive functioning (i.e., planning, organiz-
            ing, sequencing, abstracting)

B. The cognitive deficits in Criteria A1 and A2 each cause significant im-
    pairment in social or occupational functioning and represent a signifi-
    cant decline from a previous level of functioning.

C. The course is characterized by gradual onset and continuing cognitive
    decline (APA 1994).

This definition contains several important components. First, the deficits are *acquired.* That is, they occur in a person who has already achieved adult status, acquired adult skills, and filled adult roles. That person has and retains, despite the illness, the self-image of an adult. Although the person is now losing the skills that supported adult func-tions, her "adult" sense of self is not altered. It must be recognized and respected if any kind of positive relationship is to develop or be maintained.

An interesting study, described at the October 1996 Alzheimer Dis-ease International conference in Jerusalem, asked patients with demen-tia to complete a personality profile on themselves. Their families were asked to complete two such profiles on their loved ones, one as they were at that time and the other as they were before the onset of the illness. The patients' perceptions of themselves corresponded consistently with their families' reports of their premorbid personalities (Lahav et al. 1996).

Imagine the reaction of a retired bank manager, a private, refined gentleman, used to being treated with deference by his staff and family, now unable to control his emotional outbursts and in a personal care situation among people who are unfamiliar with his background and nature. Imagine his efforts to cope with being called by his first name and hearing reference made in public to his bodily functions. He might become irate, indignant, and insist that the responsible person be disci-plined or even fired. He might be described as verbally or physically "aggressive." Taken out of context, his behavior would appear irrational and "inappropriate." Understood from his perspective, however, it is not altogether unreasonable.

The second important element of the definition refers to the persistence of the condition: it does not go away. Even though the person may do better from one time to another, or under certain circumstances, the disability remains. We may be able to create the supports that enable the person to function quite well, or circumstances might simply come together. When the supports are removed or the favorable circumstances dissipate, the function once again declines. A person who is able to carry on pleasant conversation over tea served in a quiet room with only two or three other people at the table, may not even be able to glance up from his plate while trying to manage a meal of meat and potatoes on a full-course tray service in a noisy dining room.

Because the disability is hidden, locked away in the cranium, and because many people with Alzheimer's disease retain the social habits and skills they have acquired over a lifetime, it is easy for caregivers to forget that this person is operating under severe constraints. It is easy to expect operations, insights, and understanding that exceed the person's real abilities. One intelligent, but obviously overtaxed, daughter once threw up her hands during a discussion in her counselor's office, exclaiming, "*I* know he has a memory problem. You don't have to tell *me* about his memory problem. *You* explain it to *him,* because I keep trying to tell him and he just won't remember!"

Our expectations can also be quite inconsistent, once again because of the hidden nature of the disability. Every caregiver has, no doubt, found himself at one time or another explaining at length to a cognitively impaired person why he must be restricted in some activity, such as going out alone or smoking unattended. Usually, the more the person resists the restriction, the more elaborate the explanations become. Eventually the caregiver realizes that, if the person were able to understand and agree with the explanation, he would also have the judgment, insight, and other skills needed to go out alone, smoke a cigarette, or whatever else. Each time such a misalignment of abilities and expectations occurs, the relationship between the person and the caregiver is challenged. Even though the person might not remember the incident, the caregiver still feels guilty, resentful, or simply stressed. The key is to learn how to appraise the person's actual abilities so that our expectations will be more realistic and the necessary supports more often in place.

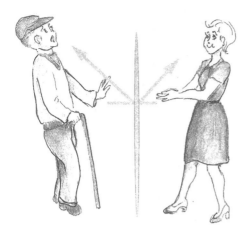

Dementia can act as a filter that distorts the person's perception of things around him and also distorts his intended actions.

The third important element refers to the pervasive nature of the illness. Dementia represents a mammoth loss to the person, cutting across every aspect of daily life. In the absence of any physical disability, the person is unable to plan a wardrobe, cook a meal, balance a checkbook, and, later, as the disease progresses, dress, bathe, or even feed himself. It is a global loss, caused by deficits in all areas of cognitive function, not just the memory that is most often cited. Very often, a functional loss or behavioral manifestation is due not to one specific cognitive impediment but to the interplay among multiple deficits. For example, a person with only poor memory is able to compensate by paying better attention; a person with poor memory and attention deficits cannot.

Dementia acts as a filter that affects both incoming and outgoing information. It distorts the impression that the person receives of the world and also the way in which his reactions are expressed.

A notion that can seriously threaten respect and, consequently, the relationship is embedded in the term *confusion*. *Confusion* is an overused, often misused, and even potentially dangerous term that describes a combination of behaviors suggesting some impairment of mental function. It is not very useful as a term in dementia care because, although it may be describing behavior due to dementia, it may also be describing behavior due to delirium, change in living conditions, or some other disruption. It is far too often used to label behavior that the caregiver does not understand. Having thus labeled the behavior, the caregiver is inclined to stop trying to understand its cause. The danger is that the behavior is simply accepted as a manifestation of dementia.

This is an example of how the notion of seeking the *rational* roots of a person's behavior is so valuable. We stop perceiving the source of the problem as being within the person. Instead, we acknowledge that the source of the problem is the lack of fit between the person's abilities and needs and the environment's capacity to accommodate them. We cannot adjust the person, and should not even try. We can and must, therefore, adjust the environment. This issue is treated in more depth in Chapter 6.

Another danger potentially associated with the word *confused* occurs when it is used to describe one person's subjective interpretation of another person's rational behavior while not fully aware of the circumstances. I once intercepted a very elderly gentleman at the nursing home door who told me that he was in a rush to go and see his mother. Fortunately, my efforts to ensure the safety of this apparently "confused" gentleman did not cause him to miss the cab that was waiting to take him to his mother's 107th birthday party. Who was the confused one here?

The Consequences of Cognitive Deficits

The exact nature of cognitive losses differs among the various dementing illnesses, and the effects of these losses will vary from person to person. What follows is not a scientific description of the nature and course of cognitive deficits associated with Alzheimer's disease but, rather, a general review of the most likely functional and behavioral consequences of the most common cognitive impairments. Suggestions for compensatory and supportive techniques and practices will be found in Chapter 6 and Chapter 8, and scattered throughout the rest of the book. What follows here is intended to give the reader a clearer impression of the situation with which the cognitively impaired person is likely to be coping and to offer some insight into that person's reactions.

When reviewing the functional consequences of losses in each of these areas, we must remember that the person's behavior is not only the result of missing or altered functions. It is evidence of the individual's efforts to continue meeting personal needs while trying to cope with, or compensate for, the changes in abilities. Just as a person riding a bicycle with defective gears might push harder and shift more often than he used to just to keep moving, the person living with a defective memory will try harder and ask questions more frequently just to stay in touch. Neither the person on the bicycle nor the cognitively impaired individual might realize exactly what is wrong. Neither might actually be aware of the exact nature of the efforts he is making. Both know that they are simply trying to make things work for them. What we see is the change in their behavior.

This chapter looks at various cognitive functions and the consequences of their impairment. The breakdown is somewhat arbitrary, however, in that our system works as a whole and the influence of one function is difficult to tease out from the influence of another. For example, memory is affected by attention. If one does not notice something, one is not likely to remember it. Perception is affected by memory. If one does not hold the details of a situation in memory long enough to put it together, one cannot perceive the whole situation accurately. Memory also affects insight. If one does not remember a situation and how it came about, how can one have insight into it? What follows, therefore, is a working model, not a definitive description.

Memory Loss

Everyone has, at one time or another, misplaced keys, forgotten names, and missed appointments. It is stressful and frightening, but in no way does it approach the experience of a person with memory loss. A forgetful or absentminded person knows what he has forgotten. No matter how frustrating it might be, he can employ a variety of mechanisms to jog his memory. He can make an active effort to recall. When he is reminded, he recognizes the material for which he was searching. A cognitively impaired person, on the other hand, frequently is not even aware that he has forgotten, does not recognize that he has a memory loss, and so is repeatedly confronted with events and circumstances for which he is unable to account.

The memory loss, or *amnesia,* of Alzheimer's disease usually affects recent memories, that is, the recollection of events that occurred moments, days, or months ago. The memory of events in the distant past is usually preserved well into the latter stages of the illness. Memory loss of this kind results in:

- difficulty acquiring new knowledge;
- disorientation to place, time, and person;
- repetitive questioning;

- paranoid ideation and confabulation; and
- anxiety and lack of insight.

Let's examine each of these consequences in more detail.

The inability to acquire new knowledge makes it difficult for the person to learn new tasks, gain new skills, and change old habits. Caregivers often report that the cognitively impaired person persists in applying old familiar rules or skills to new games. At Day Away, the day program described in *Doing Things* (Zgola 1987), one lady, a veteran golfer, continued to try applying her golfing skills to the new game of croquet. We only had to convince her that the croquet mallet was more like a putter than a driver.

Another example of difficulty acquiring new knowledge and shedding old habits occurred when a gentleman, newly admitted to a retirement home, apparently started making inappropriate sexual advances toward one of the female residents. Virtually every night he was found climbing into bed with her. Queries with his family confirmed that this was entirely out of character. What did come to light, however, was that his bedroom at home was to the right of the bathroom door. In the new surrounding, his bedroom was to the left, whereas the lady in question occupied the room to the right. He was simply following his old habit when returning to bed after using the bathroom.

The inability to acquire new knowledge also makes it difficult for the person to learn from experience and to adjust to new circumstances. One very useful capacity that human beings have is to adapt to whatever circumstances they find themselves in. This is a direct outcome of learning from experience. This capacity makes it possible for us to survive and even thrive under less than ideal conditions. Although we may initially be unhappy with a new situation, we quickly learn the ropes, discover and remember the best ways of doing things, and eventually know our way around. We learn how to avoid hurtful situations, or at least make the best of them. We learn where and how to find gratification and pleasure. Things finally stop feeling so bad and may even start to feel good. A person with memory loss, however, does not adjust so easily. She continues to live with the "new to this place" feeling for a long time. If that feeling is an unhappy one, the person will continue feeling unhappy in a new setting for far longer than we might have anticipated.

The capacity to comply with instructions also depends on our being able to acquire new information. We must remember the instructions for as long as it takes to complete the task. If a person's memory span does not exceed one minute, it is not likely that she will be able to sit and wait longer than that before getting up and doing something else. "Sit here and wait" is, therefore, probably one of the most futile things one can say to a memory-impaired person.

Disorientation to time, place, or person is yet another painful consequence of memory loss. The individual is unable to retain orienting information. We have all had that horrible feeling of being acutely disoriented. It might happen when you wake up from an unaccustomed nap and have no idea what time of day it is. It may come on as you desperately try to remember where you parked the car when, in fact, you took the bus to work that morning. It could be the panic that you feel as someone comes toward you, arms outstretched and smile beaming, while you desperately try to recall who this person is. Our experience with disorientation is fleeting and mercifully rare, yet we can all relate to the distress associated with being out of touch.

Given this distress, then, is it any wonder that whenever some information does come her way, the cognitively impaired person tries desperately to hold onto it? She uses a mechanism that can drive those around her crazy—repeating a question over and over again. It is the same mechanism that we use to "carry" a telephone number in our head from the phone directory to the dial pad, *working memory*. We repeat it over and over until we have finished dialing, then we promptly forget it. If anything happens that interferes with the repetition, or if we have to redial it, the number is gone and we must look it up again—in other words, repeat the question. This is exactly what a person with short-term memory loss does. She keeps the item in working memory until for some reason she drops it. Sensing that it is gone, but unable to retrieve it herself, she asks for help by repeating the question. If we understand this mechanism, we realize that "I just told you that" is yet another of those futile statements that can only create unhappiness in the relationship. Although repetitive questioning can drive a caregiver crazy and, if allowed to, can take a severe toll on the relationship, it is only the cognitively impaired person's desperate effort to cope. It is evidence of her resolute struggle to keep things in place and preserve a sense of control. Once we understand repetitive questioning for what it truly is, we can respect the person's effort instead of becoming irritated with it. We then simply repeat the information with the clarity and regard that the person needs.

Irritation with repetitive questioning comes mainly from our unconscious expectation that the person will remember. We do many things each day without expecting them to stay done. We make beds, wash dishes, shovel snow, and mow lawns, knowing full well that they will soon have to be done again. It might be hard work, but it is not frustrating or exasperating because our expectations are realistic. In this way too, we must realign our expectations of the person with memory loss. We tell her whatever she needs to know with the expectation that we may have to repeat the information many, many times. Generous and calm repetition of information, as the person seeks it, is to the cognitively impaired person what a lifesaver is to someone who is drowning. It represents solace and safety, rescue from the mire of disorientation. It contributes immensely to the atmosphere of security in which a trusting relationship can thrive. Consistency, comfortable routine, and courteous repetition will do a great deal to help overcome the problems mentioned above. They also help the person acquire new habits by exploiting the kind of memory function that most cognitively impaired persons retain, that is, *procedural memory,* which is discussed in more detail in Chapter 7.

We see another effect of short-term memory loss when a person attempts to account for current circumstances using old knowledge. This is called *confabulation.* The person may not remember the recent events that led to the present situation, but does know that things should make sense and so attempts to make a reconciliation. These efforts sometimes create situations that are confounding and even hurtful to a caregiver. The person appears to be lying or making up tales or accusing others of bizarre and unreasonable acts. This behavior can look very spiteful and manipulative. Especially if the person has a history of having been capricious or vindictive, caregivers are inclined to interpret this behavior as simply a continuation of a habitual pattern. They respond as one would normally with a person whose behavior is purposeful and who can be held accountable for its consequences. When the person's stories do not make sense, they want to explain the facts to her and help her see reason. When the accusations cause pain, the caregiver's impulse is to defend herself or ask, "How can you say that? Don't you know that I care for you and would never do that to you?" Once the mechanisms behind confabulation and paranoid ideas are understood, however, and caregivers realize that the person no longer has the memory, planning skills, and insight to be purposefully spiteful and manipulative, they can save themselves the pains of explanations and questions. In any event, because the person is unlikely to understand these explanations and questions, they serve only to undermine the relationship.

Confabulation frequently happens in response to a caregiver's open-ended question. Follow, for example, the memory-impaired person's cascade of thoughts that might ensue from a simple question such as "What did you have for breakfast?"

> I don't remember breakfast.
>
> The only logical reason why an intelligent person such as myself would not remember breakfast is that I have *not* had breakfast.
>
> Now that you mention it, I do not recall any meals in this place, so I think that they do not have meal services here.
>
> I haven't eaten for a long time.

So the answer comes out, "They don't serve breakfast here. It was nice talking to you, but I think I'll be going home now. I'm getting hungry. Good-bye."

Accusations and paranoid ideas result from a similar process. Mrs. K., now living in a long-term care facility, has been accusing the staff and other residents of stealing her watch. This is how things might have evolved:

> Over the past few years, Mrs. K. has experienced numerous losses: her home, the china, the mahogany furniture, her fur coat, her friends, simply too many to mention. Among the precious belongings she still has is the watch her father gave her when she graduated from nursing school. (The watch in question could be the original or it could simply have the significance of the original. That is immaterial.) Her habit is to put it on the soap dish when she washes her hands. That is normal. But is it wise to display such a precious piece in a place where so many losses have already occurred? So, being a sensible woman, she tucks it away somewhere safe as she washes her hands, but immediately forgets. Of course, she also forgets that she has forgotten and remembers only that she always puts the watch on the soap dish. The only reasonable conclusion, then, when she looks in the soap dish and discovers that it is gone, is that one of the people whom she has seen going by took it.

Care providers encounter many baffling and hurtful accusations from clients with memory loss and must be prepared to trace these accusations to their origin instead of simply yielding to the impulse of self-defense. One very common accusation comes from the female client with Alzheimer's disease who insists that the in-home care worker is having an affair with her husband. Let's just follow the line of reasoning that might lead the client to this conclusion:

I did not and never would hire a cleaning lady.

I am, after all, a competent, efficient homemaker and a frugal woman.

There is a woman coming into my house doing things that make me uncomfortable.

I cannot see any earthly reason for her coming here because I have always done my own housework and done it very well, too.

I feel threatened.

The most serious threat that I could imagine would be the loss of my greatest source of security, my husband.

That is why she makes me so uncomfortable—she is after my husband.

Given the implications of memory loss as they have been described here, is it any wonder that memory loss is so often accompanied by anxiety and what we call "lack of insight"? Imagine not knowing how you got here, where you are to go next, what is expected of you, and how you will get home—to that comfortable place where things are familiar. Imagine you are surrounded by people whom you do not recognize but who all seem to know you. They also seem to know things about you that you do not recall having told to anyone. You do not recollect when things changed and why, but you are intelligent enough to know that things were different at one time. You were busy, respected, and comfortable.

How "appropriate," by conventional standards, do you think your behavior might be under such circumstances? Effective care comes from understanding the origins of a person's feelings and hence her behavior, acknowledging the validity of those feelings, and then enlisting techniques that will address those feelings positively. Details of this approach are discussed in Chapters 6 and 8. The first step, however, comes in the effort to truly appreciate what this person might be experiencing.

Language Deficits

The technical aspects of language deficits and various options for coping with them are more fully explained in Chapter 9. What follows here is a short overview of the problem. To understand *aphasia,* language deficits, we must first distinguish *language* from *speech.* Speech is the ability to articulate words, whereas language is the ability to encode ideas into words and decode ideas from words. Speech, which is a function of muscle coordination in the throat and mouth, is seldom affected by dementias such as Alzheimer's disease. Language, on the other hand, is very often compromised by dementing illness. Language has two basic components, receptive and expressive. *Receptive language* refers to the ability to decode and, therefore, understand the ideas of others; *expressive language* refers to the ability to encode and, therefore, express one's own ideas. Although they may not be affected to the same extent, both receptive and expressive language are usually compromised to some degree.

Disruption of receptive language ability may make it difficult for the person to recognize words and understand complex sentences. When we are experiencing a communication problem with a cognitively impaired individual, we must determine whether it is the meaning of the word that is eluding him or whether he is failing to conceive the idea. This is an important distinction. If the person is having difficulty with the word, it might help to use a synonym or to describe the article and so help him grasp what you are saying. If, on the other hand, the person is having difficulty conceptualizing the idea, no matter how many synonyms you use he will not grasp your meaning. The ability to conceive abstract ideas is discussed further in this chapter. In any event, it is good practice to support verbal communication with concrete examples or gestures, simply to give the cognitively impaired person the best chance of understanding.

A person with expressive language problems will have difficulty finding the words that express his ideas accurately, constructing meaningful sentences, and mediating actions through internal speech. He may say the wrong word, substituting either a sound-alike word or a word in the same category for the intended word. This is called *paraphasia*. He might search in vain for the word and come out with "thing-a-ma-jig" or "whatever," or simply give up. This is called *anomia*. He might also try to express the idea by talking around the intended word, providing extensive descriptions and elaboration. This is called *circumlocution*. In the early stages it can cause the person to sound grandiose and even very learned. Eventually, though, we see the person's real inability to get to the point. Another indication of expressive language problems is the inability to put words into the correct order and form a meaningful sentence. The words may tumble out in the jargon of a previous occupation or eventually deteriorate into a mass of words and near-words that is descriptively called a *word salad*. These problems can combine to create severe barriers to communication. It is very important for the caregiver to remember that the person's language may reflect not his ideas but rather only the degree to which he is able to encode those ideas into words.

Another aspect of language that affects function is the ability to mediate actions through internal speech. We normally make plans or work out a problem in our head before we take action. We generally do this with words. We "talk ourselves through" a complex task, step by step, giving ourselves feedback about our progress and plotting our next action. A person who can no longer use words effectively also loses this medium of rational planning and problem solving. His approach to a task or a problem will become impulsive and without organization or purposeful flow. He will need someone else to give him step-by-step directions and consistent and discerning feedback.

Deficits in Attention

A person who does not stay with any one task for more than a few minutes is a special challenge to caregivers. This person may not sit through a meal, may wander about the house constantly looking for something to do but engaging in nothing in particular, or may become distracted halfway through a task and go off half-dressed or half-shaven. These are the most common behavior patterns that we refer to as attention problems, but attention deficits are evident through a variety of other behaviors as well. These include:

- inability to start or stop a task or action;
- fixation on one, perhaps very peripheral, aspect of a task and forgetting the task itself;
- inability to resist distraction;
- diminished responsiveness; and
- indiscriminate responsiveness.

These problems stem from a disturbance in the person's ability to direct, focus, and maintain vigilance selectively. There is a kind of "stickiness" in the behavior of a person with attentional deficit. There are two extremes to the phenomenon, *inertia* and *perseveration*. The person may have trouble getting started on a task—as though the engine just does not catch. This is inertia. Unless the caregiver identifies and understands inertia well, he may misinterpret it as resistance and recalcitrance. A caregiver who persists in trying to reason this person into activity will succeed only in frustrating himself and the person whom he is trying to motivate. It often takes some outside force, such as a gesture or a visual or tactile prompt, to help the person initiate the action or task. Once started, this same person may be unable to stop. He may persist in the activity, be it shaving, sweeping, or whatever, until some outside force brings him to a halt. This latter tendency is perseveration.

A person with attentional problems may be unable to withstand any distraction at all. He may respond with equal intensity to all stimuli, whether they are relevant to the task or not. Unable to focus on any one stimulus, this person is torn among all the activities that are going on around him. The consequence may be that he is unable to do anything or frantically tries to respond to everything. On the other hand, he may become so immersed in one particular part of the task that he becomes totally oblivious to his surroundings. He may even lose track of the job as a whole. For example, while putting on a shirt, the person may become totally immersed in doing and undoing one button and forget all about getting dressed.

The ability to attend selectively, that is, to remain focused or to switch attention at will, is one that we also tend to take for granted because our brain does it for us automatically. Our system filters out meaningless and irrelevant stimuli until we cease being aware of them at all. The question as to what makes a stimulus meaningful and relevant enough to hold the attention of a person with cognitive impairment is the object of study among professionals who design environments and interventions for persons with Alzheimer's disease and other dementing illnesses. Dr. Dale Lund and his team at the University of Utah Gerontology Center are working with videotaped sessions that they call "Video Respite" (Lund et al. 1995). Their object was to design a videotape that would hold the attention and interest of cognitively impaired persons long enough to give the caregiver a little private time. They found that some of the tapes held the attention of subjects in the study, who normally attended no longer than five minutes, for up to fifty-five minutes. Research is continuing to determine which features of the tape enable such attentiveness. Is it that the material taps into retained abilities and memories and is therefore pertinent to the person? Is it that the pacing is slow enough to let the person digest the material, yet swift enough to sustain interest? Is it that the presentation is simple enough for the person to decipher, yet adult enough to promote comfortable participation?

These questions are yet to be explored. However, the important lesson is that it is possible to structure programs, activities, and environments that capture and exploit the capacities for attention that the person retains and that restless pacing, frenetic activity, or listless inactivity is not an inevitable consequence of Alzheimer's disease. Things can be changed. In the Tea Group described in Chapter 12, we found that women who would not stay with a meal tray for more than five minutes were able to sit over their tea and cookies comfortably for an hour. Given that demonstrated ability, could their meals not have been the same kind of experience?

We often measure attention in terms of responsiveness. We associate unresponsiveness with lack of attention. This association needs to be questioned. The assumption that the person who is unresponsive is also unaware can be very destructive to the relationship. Although it may take a greater volume of stimulation to provoke a reaction from a person who is very withdrawn, particularly in the latter stages of the dementing illness, it is dangerous to infer that a person who does not react does not feel. It could very well be that the stimulus was seen or heard but failed to hold the person's attention because it was not meaningful to him. It could also be that it held his attention but that he was unable to respond, or chose, for whatever reason, not to respond. Whatever we say or do within sight or earshot of anyone must be done with the understanding that the person is somehow registering the information. Even if the person may not be able to indicate understanding of specific words and gestures, there are many messages embedded in the tone of voice and body language that the person might be grasping. These messages must continue to convey our respect and regard for the person and support that all-important positive relationship.

The onus falls on the caregiver to seek out the reason for the person's reluctance or inability to respond. One of the most common and reversible reasons why a person with cognitive impairment might withdraw is fear. Why do we find it easy to respond in some situations and find ourselves tongue-tied and recalcitrant in others? It is usually a matter of whether or not we feel safe and comfortable. If the situation is free from threat of embarrassment, failure, or retribution, we are likely to go ahead. To illustrate: How likely is a shy person, who feels nonmusical and clumsy, to respond when asked to dance and sing in front of a large group of strangers? If we are asked to do something risky, we are more likely to accept the challenge if the atmosphere is nonjudgmental and accepting. A cognitively impaired person is no different. Much of the withdrawal, reticence and apparent inattention we see among the persons with more severe dementia is due to a fear of failure, insecurity, and discomfort. It is due to consistently excessive demands and inadequate supports within the environment. We saw this effect among the women who participated in the Tea Group described in Chapter 12. Once they knew that they would never be embarrassed, that they could not fail at anything they tried, they started to take risks, and some of their responses indicated that they had been comprehending far more than anyone had suspected. They had simply chosen not to respond, and they had done it for so long that it had become a habit.

Deficits in Insight, Judgment, and Abstraction

Deficits in insight, judgment, and abstract thinking, along with diminished control over emotional expression and appreciation of the emotional expression of others, make a cognitively impaired person appear stubborn, unrealistic, and egocentric. They can also put a tremendous strain on the caring relationship. Unless a caregiver understands the origin of such behavior, the impulse to make a cognitively impaired person see reason will lead to arguments and negative feelings. These deficits also lead to:

- refusing help because of unrealistic assessment of circumstances;
- holding onto old personal standards;
- not accepting evidence of diminished abilities;
- loss of social propriety, or disinhibition;
- impaired ability to foresee consequences;
- inability to conceive objects and circumstances that are not present; and
- a tendency to take things literally.

One of the more distressing situations that community in-home care providers face is that of a cognitively impaired person who lives at home, sometimes in filth and squalor, and despite sufficient means, fails to purchase services or even refuses them when they are offered. This person may strongly resist efforts to introduce services, even to the point where he endangers his health, yet he cannot appreciate the severity of his situation. Usually, this is a person who previously kept an acceptable household by himself. Gradually he stopped attending to matters, one after another, until those who know him became concerned. Now, because he does not perceive the changes, he cannot understand why everyone is so worried. He never accepted help in the past, and so, he refuses help now. He might even perceive efforts to introduce help as an intrusion and a threat. He might even literally barricade himself in against the intrusion and so place himself in even greater jeopardy.

On a less dramatic but equally distressing level is the person who is obviously heading for trouble with a task and becomes irate and irritable with anyone who tries to correct her. Both these situations arise because the person does not realize that things have changed and therefore cannot understand the need for unaccustomed action. Efforts to help are perceived as interference, especially if the person is already inclined to be defensive. Continued efforts to convince the person of her errors simply increase the perception of threat and contribute to antagonism. Details of dealing with this situation are discussed in Chapter 6. However, a guideline, if such a thing can be said to exist in dementia care, is to start at a mutually acceptable point of reference. Then enlist the person's remaining capacity for logical thought. Here is an example of this approach at work.

Mr. Y. was the founder of a prestigious and successful travel agency. His apartment was filled with wonderful travel mementos arranged on what must have been beautiful furniture. When Mr. Y. came to the attention of our clinic, this beautiful furniture was hardly visible under the layers of trash, unopened mail, empty grocery bags, and newspapers. He spent his days sitting in one small alcove amid the piles of stuff, smoking and watching television. He shopped for essentials and cooked himself simple meals, mostly fried eggs, sausage, and toast supplemented with fruit and frozen cakes. The only help he accepted was letting his daughter do his laundry. She had done it for the past fifteen years, since Mrs. Y. had passed away. Otherwise he would let no one clean or tidy. In fact, every visitor was told bluntly that he did not want anyone touching his private things. He was fine, had been fine all his life, and intended to stay that way. When they tried to do anything, he became very upset and even threatened violence. Concern was building that his collection of papers was becoming a fire hazard. The more intense the efforts to intervene became, the more obstinate and resistant he became.

The community caseworker had to break this cycle of perceived intrusion and defense. She came to his home and made it clear that she was simply a social visitor with no intention of imposing any service on him. He accepted this with relief. He finally had someone who just wanted to visit. With all these people coming and going, no one had just wanted to talk to him. Here was the mutually acceptable point of reference: Mr. Y. was lonely.

Now to enlist his capacity for logic. This gentleman did realize that a visitor could not be expected to stand. The caseworker asked his permission to move some of the stuff so that she could sit down. She noticed that it was mostly old newspapers, and asked him if he really needed papers that were so old. He said, "No, not really." Would he mind, then, she asked, if she just put them by the door? She could take them to the garbage chute on her way down. "Yes, that would be fine," he agreed, and seemed quite pleased with the idea. On her way out, the worker asked if there was something else she could take while she was going to the garbage room. "No," he said, she shouldn't bother. He would take the rest out later. So she left with only one bundle of newspapers. That was the start of the clearing out. Mr. Y. did not take out any of the garbage, but the caseworker did the next time she visited. Each visit she noticed something else that did not make sense to keep around. The bundles of stuff that were going to the garbage chute, with his permission, became bigger and bigger.

One day she asked if they might have a cup of coffee. She could make it. There was no room in the sink to fill the water pot, so she asked him if she could do some of the dishes. Mr. Y. was obviously taken aback by this role shift. Visitors do not usually volunteer to do the dishes. This was different, she said; he was more like a friend now, and besides, it would only take a moment. He relented, and so the first inroad into cleaning had been made. Each step was done with his permission, with his agreement that it was a sensible thing to do. Eventually Mr. Y. agreed that the place did look better and that it would be nice to keep it this way, even get some more things cleaned up. He agreed to hire a cleaning lady if the caseworker could recommend one and introduce her. This handover was very important because the approach of respectful involvement was essential to maintaining Mr. Y.'s cooperation. The transfer was successful.

There was a problem, however, in getting him to pay the agency. When the bill came, he insisted that he had not hired this woman and refused to pay. The bill was outside of the immediate, concrete context of the situation that he could comprehend. Shortly after the homemaker was hired, the community worker "noticed" several unopened pension checks and bills and suggested to him that these important papers should be seen to. His daughter had a power of attorney from the time when he was in the hospital. Maybe it was time to see if she could lend a hand with the finances. Being able to follow the logic of each step as it was presented to him and seeing that his integrity was consistently respected, Mr. Y. agreed. He was, after all, a sensible person and knew that his bills had to be paid.

Some might say that this approach was very costly. It involved a community caseworker for seven visits until the homemaker was accepted and another two visits to establish the power of attorney. Before this program, however, Mr. Y. had turned down five homemakers, each of whose visits was not only a total waste of time but also added to Mr. Y.'s defensiveness, his daughter's stress, and the frustration of the agency workers who only wanted to provide good service. The result of this intervention was that Mr. Y. remained in the community for two years, an outcome that had not been foreseen when he was first referred. The original referral anticipated that he would be moved into a care facility right away because he was unable to comply with home support services and represented a hazard to himself and others.

Perhaps the most challenging instances of an impaired person's inability to assess his own abilities while holding on to old standards of performance revolve around driving. This function is deeply associated with autonomy, efficacy, status, and role, especially among men of the generations who are now in care. When driving is no longer safe, the caregiver must make a difficult decision to have the person's license suspended and to remove access to the car. If there has been a precipitating incident, such as an episode of becoming lost or an accident that frightened the person sufficiently to stick in his memory, or if there is some physical evidence such as a dent in the car or an injury, this can serve as the mutually accepted point of reference leading to the decision to stop driving. Although the explanation might have to be repeated frequently, at least the person and his caregiver can proceed along a logical path that leads to an unpleasant, but reasonable conclusion. The explanation might sound like this:

"Remember that bump on your head, Dad?"

"Yes."

"That happened the time you hit the fire hydrant. That was really frightening, because you were always such a careful driver. Your reflexes are not what they used to be. You were lucky that it wasn't a person. I know it is hard on you, but you had better not take a chance. Please let me drive you."

If the person refuses to acknowledge any incident or if, mercifully, there has been no such incident, the mutually accepted point of reference will be harder to find. The caregiver might have to rely on the strength of the relationship and simply impose the restriction. This means laying out the reasons with authority and compassion, acknowledging the person's justified distress with the situation, and trusting that their mutual regard and trust will see them through. It is important that the person with dementia never get the impression that the restriction is being imposed because the caregiver finds him incompetent or inadequate. This can be a danger in a person whose thought processes are very concrete. If the two people have previously begun a discussion about the cognitively impaired person's memory problems (this is discussed further in Chapter 9), the illness and its consequences become the problems that they face together and the reasons for the restriction. With a problem as critical as driving, it may be necessary to take a more pragmatic approach and, if the family can function without a vehicle, simply remove the car, saying that it is out of order and beyond repair. Whatever the reason cited, everyone involved must explain it consistently.

Loss of social propriety and disinhibition comes from a failure in the filtering system that determines which thoughts we keep to ourselves, which ones we express and how we express them, which impulses we suppress and which ones we act on. The person might simply say what occurs to her without regard for the context or possible consequences. She might act out impulses that would normally never have surfaced. Often these have sexual overtones or involve some vulgarity that is alien to the person's habitual character. The person might also be inclined to give full rein to emotional expressions. She might respond to mildly amusing situations with unbridled glee or become furious over something that would normally be a trivial irritant. This behavior is a symptom of the dementing illness. It is not willful or malicious. The person cannot control it, and is usually not even aware of its inappropriate nature. Efforts to make the person accountable are likely to create even more problems, because they demand the impossible and put her on the defensive. Follow this unfortunate line of events:

> Mr. K. sits in a wheelchair. As a young woman walks by his chair, he reaches up and touches the most accessible part of her. She turns in shock and asks him why he did that. He is not aware of having done anything that should cause such a reaction. In fact, he would never do anything that might upset her like that. So why should he account for his actions? But she is obviously disturbed and angry with him. Besides, she is far too young to be talking to him that way, so he puts her in her place. He cannot filter his language and uses some coarse expression that gives the young woman even greater offense. And so a situation that started from nothing escalates.

This situation arose from Mr. K.'s inability to inhibit his impulse, his inability to foresee the consequences of his actions, and his inability to control his emotional expression. It was fueled by the visitor's normal reaction to something she did not understand. The potential for a situation such as this lurks in almost every encounter with a cognitively impaired person. It can lead to acrimony or even dangerous situations, with the person striking out or trying to run away. It is one of the reasons why the care of persons with dementia requires such vigilance. Techniques for handling these situations are discussed in more detail in Chapter 8. However, here are some guidelines:

- Recognize the behavior for what it really is, the symptom of an illness. We would not expect a person with chicken pox to take responsibility for his spots.
- Avoid questions that the person cannot answer and that put him on the spot.
- Ignore the behavior whenever possible.
- If the behavior cannot be ignored, avoid the circumstances that precipitate it, or simply tell the person that you do not like it and ask him to do you a favor by stopping it.
- Avoid arguments and efforts to reform the person.

One of the most painful consequences of this uninhibited behavior is social isolation. It is often imposed by the caregiver's embarrassment and fear of exposing the person's illness. However, many caregivers find that their friends, neighbors and other people are far more tolerant and understanding than they had anticipated. One woman had ceased bringing her husband to church because she feared that his enthusiastic singing was disturbing the congregation. She brought him back when she found out that not only was the congregation not disturbed, they actually missed him. They were pleased to know that there was something he could still enjoy so much and agreed that his participation gave a new dimension to their worship. There are times when the person's uninhibited candor can be an eye-opener. A director of nursing started a serious weight reduction plan that eventually saved his life when a disinhibited resident told him in graphic terms that his weight was a hazard not only to his own health but also to that of his wife.

The inability of a cognitively impaired person to conceive of objects that are not evident or to grasp abstract ideas often takes caregivers by surprise. If we can imagine someone actually living in a reality where "out of sight" is really "out of mind," we will have a better appreciation of the term "concrete thinking." The behavioral consequences of this disability can also be staggering.

One caregiver came to the office in distress. She had evidence that her cognitively impaired mother really did hate her after all (she had long been convinced of this). Mother and daughter, whose ages were only fifteen years apart, had lived together for some years. The daughter had severe rheumatoid arthritis and her mother had Alzheimer's disease. Mother did the heavy work in the house under her daughter's direction. The daughter was convinced that her mother's reticent and obstinate behavior was due to resentment and hate. Now she had proof! They had been sitting in the living room, watching television, when she asked her mother to make her a cup of tea. Her hands were very sore and a cup of tea would be so nice. Mother simply said, "No." The daughter could cope with that. This is simply the way that Mother had been lately, negative. She could do without the tea. However, what happened next really drove a sword through her heart. Mother got up, went into the kitchen, made herself a cup of tea, came back into the living room, sat down, and drank it in front of her. If this was not a gesture of hatred, what else could it be?

An interview with the mother revealed that she did not have the memory and planning skills needed to undertake such a complex scheme. In addition, no matter what their previous relationship might have been, she now harbored no animosity toward her daughter. What had actually happened? When her daughter asked for the cup of tea, the mother had no idea how to go about complying with the request. There were no cues for her in the living room. So she did the only thing she could do and said, "No." When she spontaneously went into the kitchen, all the tea things were there. She had all she needed to make the tea, only no clue as to how many cups to make. She was alone in the kitchen and so she made only one cup. By the time she came into the living room and drank the tea in front of her daughter, she had forgotten her daughter's request and was only doing a natural thing with no rancor or ill will.

The tendency to take things literally comes from the inability to conceptualize the abstract and can catch the caregiver unawares. It can also produce some unbelievable situations. One caregiver told of an incident where he inadvertently gave his wife an arduous task by using a figure of speech that she took literally. Each morning they sorted the mail together, filed the bills, read the correspondence and checked out the advertisements. One morning he got up leaving some flyers on the table. "What do you want me to do with these?" his wife asked him. "Just stick them in the top drawer," he answered. An hour later he found her, having removed everything from the top drawer, and meticulously lining it with the flyers and sticky tape. In another case, a woman had asked her husband to clean the street salt from the carpet in the car. She had pointed to one spot to illustrate what she wanted him to do. The one spot to which she had pointed was exactly what he cleaned and nothing else. In her exasperation she shouted at him, "Maybe I should do this myself!" "Okay," he answered and walked away from the job.

Another aspect of problems in this area is the person's impaired ability to appreciate the emotional expressions of others. Even though a caregiver may understand the origin of the behaviors as described above, the failure of the person to appreciate or respond to the caregiver's feelings is perhaps one of the greatest ordeals of giving care. "It's like living in a vacuum," said one caregiver. Caregivers dealing with such situations can be exposed to immense emotional stress. The worst of it is that there is often no overt evidence of the source of this stress. To the outside visitor, a cognitively impaired person often sounds entirely reasonable. He musters a socially appropriate or near-appropriate response when the caregiver least expects it, usually in the doctor's office. If he is somewhat disinhibited around strangers, the effect is usually amusing. Under such circumstances it is difficult for the caregiver to share feelings or even find someone who will believe what is really going on. Many caregivers in this situation would benefit from professional counseling and ongoing support. They often need encouragement to seek help and to continue seeking help until they find it.

Perceptual and Visuospatial Deficits

Distortions in perception, that is, the inability to make sense of one's senses, can affect every modality. Because we depend so heavily on vision and because our ability to interpret information coming through our eyes is so refined, deficits in visual perception have a tremendous impact on a cognitively impaired person's ability to function. Deficits in visual perception can result in:

- failure to recognize objects or people;
- misinterpreting environmental cues (illusions);
- difficulty finding things in a clutter or on a poorly contrasted background;
- tripping and inaccurate reach;
- way-finding difficulties; and
- anxiety and insecurity.

A cognitively impaired person's failure to recognize familiar objects, *agnosia,* can be perplexing. Asked to pick up his spoon, the person may look straight at it, yet fail to recognize the object in front of him as a spoon. Once it is placed in his hand, his fingers seem to remember the feel of the spoon even though his eyes have forgotten its sight, and he can use it correctly. Sometimes, however, even this back-up mechanism fails and the person cannot recognize the object in his hand or confuses it with something similar. For instance, he might try to comb his hair with a toothbrush.

The failure to recognize faces is a particular dysfunction called *apresbignosis*. One of our clients had an undiagnosed cortical illness that caused this problem. He was aware of what was happening to him and so was able to give us some insight. "I know who you are," he once told me, "because I came into your office, but when I look at you, it is as though I see you for the first time." He had to trust his memory of contexts to know who people were. Otherwise he was constantly among strangers. The problem can extend to the person's ability to recognize himself in a mirror. This gentleman would say, "I am looking into a mirror, hence the face I see must be my own, even if I do not recognize it." The person with a global dementia, though, does not recognize his own disability and therefore concludes that the face that he does not recognize must be that of a stranger.

> One gentleman had become incontinent. His wife felt that his illness had not progressed sufficiently to account directly for this and decided to investigate. Sometimes he would go outside and urinate in the backyard. At other times he would have an accident in the house. The remarkable thing was that he was never incontinent during the night. When his wife watched him closely, she saw him go to the bathroom door, open it, stop abruptly, mutter "Oh, excuse me," close the door softly and walk away. She correctly concluded that he had caught sight of himself in the bathroom mirror, thought that the room was occupied, and left. Of course, with the bathroom constantly occupied, the poor man had no alternative but to go outside. Sometimes he just didn't make it. At night he was used, from years of habit, to getting up in the dark and, of course, did not see anyone in the mirror. The simple removal of the vanity mirror solved this gentleman's incontinence problem.

Sometimes the combination of a cognitively impaired person's retained abilities, lifelong habits, needs, and disability create baffling problems.

> Miss M. had lived alone for many years in a two-roomer above a hardware store in the center of town. The store owner and some neighbors looked out for her and, despite her severe cognitive impairment, Miss M. managed adequately. People became concerned, however, when she started to lose weight. Miss M. complained frequently about a lady in her bedroom who was wearing her clothes without permission. This lady in the mirror did not threaten Miss M.'s well-being, but the people she saw coming to the window at night did. Miss M. felt sorry for them and insisted on preparing meals for them. They never ate the food and that distressed her. She had been a practi-

cal nurse and housekeeper. She had nursed her sick father single-handedly until his death. She was a caring woman who was used to putting other people's needs before her own, and that is what she now continued to do. She would put food out for the poor souls at the window instead of eating it herself. When we tried installing blinds, she simply peeked behind to see one of them staring back at her. The only solution, eventually, was to help Miss M. move into a care facility before she starved herself. Long-term care actually suited her very well. There she found many people whom she could help without putting herself in jeopardy.

When a person can no longer identify things in his environment accurately, especially if he is unaware of the fact, he is apt to experience illusions. This is due to misinterpretation of real stimuli. Shadows may appear to be figures; fluttering curtains may look like scampering creatures. This phenomenon is quite different from hallucinations. Hallucinations occur when a person's brain actually fabricates visions and sounds that have no concrete basis. Some medications, especially those taken for Parkinson's disease, may cause visual hallucinations. Otherwise, hallucinations are a rare occurrence in dementia care.

A person who has expressive language problems and also experiences illusions can pose a challenge to the caregiver. When he is upset by the "thief at the window," it could be the shadow of the curtain that looks like someone sneaking in. If you ask him whether he is referring to "that dark thing by the window," and he says yes, it is a simple matter to assure him that, although it could look like a thief, it is really a shadow and nothing to worry about. But when he looks out of the third story of his apartment building, points to a front-end loader near a group of park benches, and says that he hopes the dragon is not going to hurt the children, the caregiver has to stop and think. Has he mistaken the concrete sides of the park bench for children? Does the yellow machine look to him like a dragon? Or is this really a language problem and is he really trying to say that he hopes the front-end loader (dragon) won't take out (hurt) the park benches (children) as part of the construction that is obviously under way? Or was he thinking of something else altogether and just came up with the words from a familiar old fairy tale? Under such circumstances it is best to let the person know that you haven't understood exactly what he means but that you are prepared to figure it out with him. It is also very helpful to be aware of all the possibilities.

Another aspect of visual perception that may be compromised is the ability to distinguish an object from its background. This problem can make it difficult for a person to see silver cutlery on a white tablecloth, for example. It might obscure the white toilet in a white tiled bathroom and cause a gentleman to use the more obvious red wastebasket instead. The same problem can make it difficult for the person to spot one item in a drawer full of things, or an object set upon a complicated background. Eventually specific objects just blend into the background and discrimination is impossible for the person unless specific items are pointed out.

When a person loses the ability to judge depth and distance, the world becomes very unpredictable. Unable to judge how high or low a mark on the ground is, he is likely to step over it very carefully to make sure he clears it, or to walk all around it to avoid falling in. Without the ability to judge height, he has no way of telling that the yellow shape on the yellow carpet is a chair and likely to trip him if he tries to tread on it, while the blue shape is a design and perfectly safe to step on. Because changes in floor texture or color often represent changes in elevation, a cognitively impaired person might be led to anticipate a stair between the carpet and the linoleum. Anyone who has come down a flight of stairs, anticipating an extra stair where there was none, will know what a spine-jarring experience that can be. Stairs without clearly marked risers can be totally imperceptible. Here too a cognitively impaired person may have a painful surprise. Patterned carpets, checkered tiles, and shiny floors (which can look wet) can all make an area virtually impossible for this person to negotiate. Another potential hazard is carpeted baseboards that disguise the boundary between the floor and the wall. They create the illusion that the floor goes out another eight inches. Misjudging his distance from the wall, the person may experience some painful collisions. Furniture that obscures a clear path between two points in a room will create an impassable barrier for a person with visuoperceptual problems. The same mechanism, the inability to judge distance and depth, is at work when the person tries to reach for an object and either knocks it over or grasps at thin air, or when he puts an object down beside or in front of a table, or on top of another object.

The inability to appreciate direction and the relative position of objects to one another in space results in trouble differentiating left and right, front and back, before and behind, and so on. As a consequence the person has difficulty putting on clothes, setting the table, or finding his way in familiar surroundings. It also becomes difficult for cognitively impaired persons to adjust to new surroundings. With their world becoming so unpredictable, is there any wonder that cognitively impaired persons are apt to become anxious and insecure, especially in unfamiliar circumstances?

Deficits in Motor Organization

Most of the things we do in the course of daily living require many more steps from intent to action than we are aware of. For example, what is the first movement you make when you rise from a chair? Most people have to go through the motion before they can answer that question. Then they realize that the first thing they do is tuck their feet under the chair and shift their body weight forward. Only when their nose is well in front of their toes can they lift themselves comfortably up from the chair.

Over the years, our body's wiring system has acquired millions of movement patterns that we enlist automatically, as the need arises. Ask people who type where the letter "q" is on the keyboard and watch as they pretend to type out a word containing that letter. They will reach up high with the fifth finger of the left hand. That is the location of the letter "q" in the body's typing pattern. Many movement patterns have been so embedded that they are no longer accessible to the conscious mind. The typist has lost conscious contact with the location of letters. The body, however, remembers.

The fact that these patterns are "hardwired" into our system means that we need not think of them each time we perform a task. Our body moves smoothly through the action and all we are aware of is that the job is being done. It leaves our mind free for higher executive operations such as quality control and decision making. The function that enables us to access these patterns properly is called *praxis*. To appreciate the importance of this function, imagine having to think through the details of brushing your teeth. Imagine:

You are right-handed.

- In which hand do you hold the toothbrush?
- Which end do you grasp?
- Which hand do you use to squeeze the toothpaste? For how long?
- How do you orient the tube to the brush?

You are now holding the toothbrush in your left hand and the toothpaste in your right.

- What do you do now to comfortably brush your teeth?

You manage to put the toothpaste down, switch the brush into your right hand, and brush. Your mouth is now full of toothpaste and your right hand occupied with the brush.

■ How do you get a glass of water to rinse with?

We see now how life can become very difficult when praxic functions are disrupted. Problems can arise during the course of any multiple-step task. The person may lose access to the automatic pattern and either be unable to start the activity at all or get stuck in midcourse. If he receives a concrete clue, it may get him started. He can often proceed until something distracts him or he loses touch with the pattern. Then he needs another prompt, usually starting at the beginning of the whole pattern, to continue. A similar thing happens to us when we have trouble recalling a melody. Given the first few notes, we can continue until something interrupts us and we lose track of the tune. Then we have to start again from the beginning.

One of the problems that is most frustrating to caregivers is getting a cognitively impaired person into and out of a car. The person needs some concrete starting cue, just like the few first notes of the melody, to trigger the movement pattern. He seems to be doing well, heading for the car seat but then gets stuck halfway down. No amount of encouragement or explanation will get him to sit and swing his legs in. He needs to straighten up, walk away from the car and approach it all over again. Many women find that they have particular difficulty with their husbands, who were used to driving, getting in on the passenger side of the car. This is because the men never actually acquired an automatic pattern for getting into the right side of the car. They always got in on the left. A number of wives report that they have more success in getting their husbands to sit in the left rear seat.

The other side of this problem occurs when an automatic pattern is triggered at an inappropriate time. This has happened to everyone at one time or another. After remodeling the kitchen, we continue reaching for things in the old places. We might find ourselves halfway to the office and realize that this is the morning we were supposed to go somewhere else. The old pattern, which is no longer appropriate, is triggered by a familiar stimulus. On one occasion I was standing in the hallway at our day program, holding a coat I had just taken from one lady, when another one slipped her arms into the sleeves, as though I were holding it just for her. She finished putting it on and proceeded down the hall toward the exit.

Another aspect of praxic function is the ability to put the various steps that make up a task into the correct order. Think once again of brushing teeth and list all the steps in the correct order. Imagine the consequence, now, of confusing the order. You might end up with a mouth full of toothpaste, or you might never get the toothpaste to your mouth at all. We often see persons with this difficulty putting on their underwear over their outer clothes. At the completion of each step, the person must decide what to do next. These decisions can be very difficult for the apraxic person. He may make the wrong decision or avoid the decision altogether by either stopping or persisting in one step of the task over and over again.

Here we have reviewed the five A's of dementia:

*A*mnesia

*A*phasia

*A*ttentional deficits (along with other executive functions)

*A*gnosia

*A*praxia

Understanding dementia in terms of its functional and behavioral consequences is essential to effective care, just as an understanding of the functional consequences of heart disease is essential to the effective care of a person with a cardiac condition. "Dementia" is not to be taken as a definition of a person in terms of his deficits, but rather as an understanding of the challenges with which this person is functioning. Understanding the consequences of dementia ensures that our expectations are realistic and that our efforts to help are accurately directed.

3

Getting the Facts:
History and Personal Information

Information—accurate, current, and fluid—is essential to establish, maintain, and support a relationship with the cognitively impaired person. Because the person is unable to provide and update that information independently and spontaneously, the caregiver's responsibility is to be constantly alert. An insatiable curiosity about the person's past, current experiences, abilities, and so on, is an essential characteristic of the effective caregiver. In this and the next two chapters we look at information from a variety of perspectives: personal information regarding history and personality traits that determine, to a great measure, how the person reacts; ongoing appraisal of the person's cognitive abilities; and functional assessment that evaluates not only what the person can and cannot do but also how he enlists retained abilities to get things done and where he is stymied by lost abilities.

One of the perversities of old age is that it makes people look more and more alike at a time when they are more different from one another than they have ever been. Hair color, style of dress, height, and shape all become more homogenous as the people actually become more individual. Programs for persons with Alzheimer's disease and related illnesses accommodate people ranging in age from sixty to ninety-five. That is a span of almost two generations. Could any single program hope to accommodate people ranging from twenty-five to sixty? Consider the variety of backgrounds that such a group represents and the variety of roles that they have filled. Consider also the difference that sixty to ninety-five years of life experience makes in forming memories, values, habits, prejudices, and interests. Responsive care must recognize and accommodate these differences. This is especially true in the care of persons who are unable to volunteer much information. Professional caregivers must acknowledge the individuality of their program participants or residents and constantly seek to round out their knowledge of each person's life and times. Family caregivers must also realize the value of such information, even seemingly trivial items, and bring it to the attention of the staff.

The social and historical information that is collected upon admission to any program or facility may seem adequate at the time. But it is usually given in one block at a stressful time when its relevance is not obvious to staff who have not yet had any experience with the person. We are dealing with some eighty to ninety years of living. How could one form or questionnaire suffice to identify all the information that a caregiver needs to promote a sense of security, inclusion, affection, and control in the person? We must know whether the aphasic, frail gentleman we are dealing with was a scholar or a bodybuilder, or perhaps both. If we ever hope to understand why an elderly lady becomes distressed and wants to go downstairs before settling into bed each night, we must know the circumstances of her life. We must know that she cared for her developmentally delayed sister and tucked her in every night for forty years.

To be really useful, such information must come in a variety of media and on an ongoing basis. The most effective way is to encourage staff members to maintain ongoing contact with families and ask questions. It is a good policy to involve families in regular meetings at which one of the agenda items is to clarify some items of historical information. Another way of encouraging families to provide vital information is to suggest that they become involved in the program. They might, for example, decorate the person's room with significant personal belongings, articles such as pictures, trophies, or medals that represent important events or roles in the person's life. They can prepare a photo album in which the pictures are labeled, and make it available to staff and volunteers who spend time with the person.

The staff of long-term care facilities and day programs are often shy about asking personal questions. They frequently feel that they do not have the time, responsibility, permission, or even skill to dig out such information. The residents themselves are usually able to provide very little. What follows is an exercise intended either to provoke thought about how well we really know the persons for whose quality of life we are responsible, or to be used as an actual training exercise. As an exercise, it is intended to give staff members the time, the mandate, and the tools to obtain and share personal information and history about individual residents.

Getting to Know You: A Staff Awareness Activity

This program invites participants to reflect on the importance of really knowing about the people in their care and to practice the skills needed to gather information. It consists of two components—classroom exercises and a field component—and can be broken into as many small modules as the trainer wishes.

In the classroom exercise, staff members discuss the kind of information that they would want their caregiver to have about themselves were they ever to find themselves in a dependent state. They also determine where and how such information about a person in care would most likely be obtained. This might be through direct conversation or, if the person cannot speak, by communication with family and other visitors, or by consulting community records, history books, and libraries. Staff become aware of how vital this kind of information is to their ability to care for residents, and learn to identify appropriate sources of such information.

In the field component, staff members first practice gathering information by approaching one of their own family members or friends. Having gained some experience with the process, they then collect as much information as they can about a selected resident over a given period of time. They make appointments with visitors, have individual time for interviewing the resident, or even visit the library. Each becomes an expert on the life and times of a given resident and presents this information to the rest of the team.

Part 1. What Do We Want to Do Here?

Part 1 can be used alone as a stimulus for staff members at all levels, including administrators and supervisors, to start thinking about gathering information in general. The objective is to highlight the need to learn about the individual who is dependent on others and to identify a variety of ways in which useful information can be gathered.

Introduce the topic with a discussion. The combination of cognitive impairment and new situations (such as admission to day care or an institution) often has the unfortunate effect of obliterating information about the individual's past, his or her accomplishments, failures, habits, values, hopes, fears, roles, strengths, and weaknesses. This information is essential to our ability to provide our residents with an optimum quality of life.

Let's take a moment to see how important this information really is. If you were being admitted to a long-term care facility, what would you want your caregivers to know about you? How would you feel living with and being cared for by people who did not know this? Imagine the consequences of being called by your nickname and hating it each time, or not having your bed made the way you want it, or having to sleep with a night-light when you are used to sleeping in the dark.

Does our program or facility have the means of collecting the following information about participants? If not, would it be possible to start collecting this information now? If this information is available, how is it being applied in the individual's care?

Pass out the personal information exercise (Exhibit 1).

Part 2. Staff Members Get to Know Each Other

The objective is to introduce participants (staff members) to the concept that personal information is more than just demographics. The exercise demonstrates the impact that sharing such information can have on relationships.

The leader introduces the session as a way of learning a little more about each other and looking at how such knowledge can affect the way we feel about each other and work together, both among ourselves and with the residents. Discuss examples of how, when we first meet a person, we might feel a certain way about him and make some assumptions from the way he looks or acts. Once we get to know something more about that person, however, we find we might have things in common or we just understand him better because we know a little more about his background.

The leader asks if participants know each other. The likely answer is "yes." Ask them to try to recall what, if any, musical instrument each of their colleagues plays. Then ask for the answer and see by show of hands how many were right about everyone. Do the same exercise using "What city did you grow up in?" or "What is your favorite hobby?" "Now how well do you think you know your colleagues?" "Let's get to know one another a little better."

Pass out the staff questionnaire (Exhibit 2). Go over one question at a time, and encourage participants to share the information with the group. Assure people that they need share only as much information as they wish. Have fun with it.

Ask each person to reflect on how knowing each of these little bits of information has affected their feelings toward the person to whom it pertains. Do you feel that you have something in common with this person? Share these reflections.

EXHIBIT 1. A PERSONAL INFORMATION EXERCISE

History (achievements, failures, fondest memories, interests, etc.)

Your information: _____

Is such information collected about participants? _____

How? _____

How is it used? _____

Habits (personal grooming, rituals, dress, food preferences, etc.)

Your information: _____

Is such information collected about participants? _____

How? _____

How is it used? _____

Values (work habits, racial prejudices, etc.)

Your information: _____

Is such information collected about participants? _____

How? _____

How is it used? _____

Fears (loss of money, loss of independence, the dark, etc.)

Your information: _____

Is such information collected about participants? _____

How? _____

How is it used? _____

Strengths (special skills and talents)

Your information: _____

Is such information collected about participants? _____

How? _____

How is it used? _____

Weaknesses (temper, etc.)

Your information: _____

Is such information collected about participants? _____

How? _____

How is it used? _____

EXHIBIT 2. STAFF INFORMATION FORM: GETTING TO KNOW ME

My information:	Where could someone find this out?
My nickname is _____	_____
The best thing about me is _____	_____
I was born in _____	_____
I lived most of my life in _____	_____
What was it like? _____	_____
My favorite job was _____	_____
The most influential person in my life was _____	_____
In my family I have felt closest to _____	_____
The best decision I ever made was _____	_____
My favorite thing to do is _____	_____
My favorite food is _____	_____
My favorite sport is _____	_____
My favorite place is _____	_____
Something you can always find in my refrigerator _____	_____
I am most proud of _____	_____

Ask participants to reflect on how it feels when others know these things about them. Would they feel a little more comfortable in the care of a person who knows something about them, their history, their likes and dislikes? Share these reflections.

Briefly discuss possible sources of this information in the event that the resident is not able to convey it personally. For example, ask family and friends about the times, such as wars, etc., that the person lived through. Stress that to get information you must go after it. It may not be easy. We need to practice first.

Part 3. Practice Gathering Information

This section introduces participants to the idea of actively seeking information about a person. It gives them the opportunity to identify and cope with whatever problems might come up in a less-threatening context.

EXHIBIT 3. RESIDENT INFORMATION FORM: GETTING TO KNOW YOU

Resident's name _____

Nickname _____

Believes the best thing about him/her is _____

Was born in _____

Lived most of his/her life in _____

What was it like? _____

His/her favorite job was _____

The most influential person in his/her life was _____

His/her favorite thing to do is _____

His/her favorite food is _____

His/her favorite place is _____

Other

_____

_____

_____

_____

_____

_____

Ask each participant to identify a person with whom they are comfortable but not intimately familiar, to use as a practice subject for the upcoming exercise.

Hand out the resident questionnaire (Exhibit 3). Ask them to review the questions and identify those to which they do not know the answers about the person whom they have chosen. Ask what other questions they might identify that would help them form a better relationship with that person.

Set them the tasks of (1) verifying the information that they think they already know, and (2) getting the new information. Discuss alternative ways of getting the information if the person is unable to answer directly.

Tell them that you will be arranging individual meetings with each of them to discuss progress and problems.

Part 4. Gathering Information

This section gives staff members the opportunity to use some of the insights and experiences they have gained from the exercise in Part 3, to identify the kinds of information that would be helpful to them in their interactions with residents, and to discuss the techniques they will try in obtaining it.

Obtain feedback from the practice exercise.

Hand out your new resident questionnaire. Review the questions already in place and obtain confirmation from participants that they are useful and appropriate.

Ask for suggestions of additional questions. If none are forthcoming, offer the following suggestions:

- What is the person's original language?
- How far did she reach in school?
- What kind of music does she enjoy? Play?
- Does she hold any prejudices? Racial? Religious?

Help the group identify a potential source for each of the items on the questionnaire. Other staff might be good sources as well. Direct the staff to collect, over the next two weeks, as much of the information as possible and be prepared to present the outcome of their efforts at the next group session. Let them know that they are expected to take work time to do this. Suggest appropriate times of the day when they might schedule appointments with families or chat with the resident.

Acknowledge that in some cases the information may be difficult or impossible to obtain. Make sure participants understand that they will not be judged on the nature or quantity of their information, or the quality of their presentation. Reassure them that they are among colleagues and it is the experience that counts.

Part 5. Feedback

In this session, staff members share the information they have collected. By now they have each become an expert on a particular resident's life and times. They now have an opportunity to demonstrate that expertise and perhaps present a new side of the resident whom they have researched.

Ask participants how they felt about the exercise, whether they were able to get as much information as they wanted. Discuss generally some of the successes or frustrations they may have experienced.

Invite volunteers to start the presentations. If none are forthcoming, choose the individuals who seem to have been the most at ease with the earlier exercises.

Reinforce the understanding that they are not being judged by the amount or nature of the information they have. Even if they have succeeded in obtaining very little, they have an experience to share.

Ask participants whether their understanding and impression of the resident they researched has changed, and if so, how.

Discuss procedures that can be changed or initiated as a result of the information gleaned from this experience.

Thank participants for their contributions to the ongoing evolution of the program.

Get It from the Source That Really Counts

In our search for information, we readily acknowledge that the most important person is the client. Yet the person most often overlooked as a source of information is also the client. The vast majority of admission forms to long-term care or day programs are completed by relatives, the family doctor, and the social worker responsible for the admission. Few, if any, include a section for the client to complete.

How many of us can truly say that we know our parents fully? The average child's knowledge of his parents takes him back only to the parent's mid-thirties. He knows of the parent's behavior but what does he know of the motivations behind that behavior? For example, many adult children report that their mother was an excellent cook. The activities coordinator includes this information on the lady's interest inventory and schedules her for cooking group. Who asks whether this lady really wants to cook? Perhaps she did it only for her family and is now glad to be done with it. How many of us know of our parents' dreams and aspirations when they were in high school, or the talents that they might have put aside in favor of sensible jobs and family obligations?

Most people have both public and private faces. The person who overcame shyness in order to do well in business often remains a shy person inside. The restrained lady may have been holding back an exuberant, life-of-the-party personality. Insight into this private side of a person must come directly from that person.

It is likely that by the time a cognitively impaired person is in need of special programs, he is not able to handle long and complex forms. This is really not a reason to exclude the most important person and the holder of the most valuable information from the process. Forms need not be complex and lengthy to be informative. Written forms are not the only way to collect valuable information. The investigators in the Israeli study mentioned in Chapter 2 used a list of pairs of adjectives. The person was asked to choose from each pair the adjective that best described her. They found that persons with even severe cognitive impairment were able to provide a fairly complete profile of themselves. Verbal reporting is invaluable. One of the most useful questions I consistently ask new clients is, "If someone were to tell me the best thing about you, what would they say?" I am always impressed with the insight that the answers from even very impaired individuals offers. I have had answers such as "Never late a day on the job," "You could always count on her to help," or even "Nothing much." They all provide valuable information.

When there is a discrepancy between the family's report and the person's self-report of historical information, there are two possibilities: either the family is mistaken or things have somehow been altered in the person's memory. Whatever the cause of the discrepancy, however, the person's perspective is the one that should determine programming. Unless the person has the opportunity to share that perspective, whatever it might be, an important component is missing from the whole information-gathering process.

4

Ongoing Appraisal
of the Person's Cognitive Abilities

Although initial and regular assessment for the purposes of diagnosis, monitoring, and care planning is the domain of specialists, everyone who is expected to work with the cognitively impaired person, whether offering recreational activities or helping with activities of daily living (ADLs), must have a realistic idea of the person's abilities. This comes from having access to the information gleaned through the formal assessment along with the ability to judge, on an ongoing basis, changes in the person's memory, language, perception, attention, motor planning, and other higher cognitive processes. Without such information and sensitivity, caregivers inadvertently place the person into situations that are frustrating, defeating, and destructive to the relationship. It would be a foolish baseball coach who attempts to assemble a team without some idea of whether his players can run, catch, or throw. Yet far too many care providers and family caregivers offer activities or express expectations without any clear understanding of the person's basic abilities.

One facilitator was observed conducting an activity with several elderly residents of a nursing home. For some reason, he was attempting to have participants identify the color of the clothing worn by the person next to them. One lady, looking at the blue sweater of her neighbor, tried several words: black, beige, brown. Each time she was patiently told that she was wrong and was encouraged to try again. Finally she gave up in frustration. As the session progressed, it became more and more apparent that this lady had a severe language deficit, aphasia. In search of the word *blue,* she had said every "b" color she could think of. Because of his ignorance of this lady's aphasia, the facilitator was inadvertently, yet persistently, cruelly and needlessly exposing her to failure and frustration.

A nurse was describing one of his residents as a man who needed a firm hand. "You just have to let him know who is boss," he said. "Just don't let him get away with anything. For instance," he explained, "getting Harry to dress is a simple matter of being firm. When I see him in the hall in his pajamas, I tell him, 'Harry go into your room and get your clothes on.' Harry usually will say 'no' or 'later,' but I keep at him. So I take him into his room and say again, 'Harry get dressed.' Harry's stubborn, you know, and he will usually resist that too. So I open the closet, show him his clothes and tell him again. But he's tough. I then put his clothes on the bed and give him the order again. Usually I have to pick up the clothes and hand them to him directly. Then he puts them on. You see, Harry needs a firm hand."

The relationship between Harry and the nurse could have been pleasant instead of punitive. Both of them could have been saved a great deal of strife if the nurse had understood Harry's limited ability to organize and execute a complex task such as dressing. Harry needed step-by-step, concrete cues. When the nurse eventually gave him one item of clothing at a time, Harry was able to get dressed. He would have done it willingly and happily from the start had the necessary help been available.

The following guide for ongoing appraisal of cognitive abilities does not replace or duplicate a thorough cognitive evaluation. It does not produce a diagnosis, nor even a standard assessment of the person's level of impairment. It is not an assessment tool. It does, however, give a snapshot of certain aspects of the person's cognitive ability. It describes a process of inquiry that will give the caregiver a more realistic impression of how well the person is likely to deal with situations that challenge memory, attention, language, etc. It is also useful in helping caregivers account for a cognitively impaired person's failure to achieve certain activities. When we see a person unable to follow a simple written instruction such as "clap your hands" despite being able to read it aloud, we know why she does not heed the notes we leave on the refrigerator. When we see that the person cannot recall the three words that were said to her just two minutes ago and, in fact, does not even remember having heard any particular words at all, we realize how futile it is to tell her to sit right here and wait till you get back. Only when we appreciate the true nature of the person's abilities and disabilities can we distinguish between "can't" and "won't." Sometimes it takes an objective look at the challenges that the person is facing to give the caregiver a real appreciation of the effort that the person is already making.

A word of caution about any kind of testing or inquiry into a vulnerable person's abilities is necessary here. Any activity or interaction that is likely to confront the person directly with her disability must be undertaken with sensitivity and care. The danger of asking open-ended questions, challenging a person's recent memory, or asking her to do things at which she is not likely to succeed has already been discussed. These are all invitations to failure and threats to the trusting relationship. As much as possible, try to get information about the person's abilities by observing her reactions to normally occurring situations. If you choose to investigate a skill by posing a question or a task, always prepare a way for the person to save face in the event that she is not able to manage it. For example, instead of simply asking a person to do a drawing by saying, "Can you draw this?" you might invite the person to join you in a drawing game. That way she can back out if she becomes uncomfortable. Do not embark on any direct sampling of skills unless you are confident that you can handle the person's failure in a way that will be comfortable for both of you. I once asked a former teacher to write her name for me. She did not even know how to start. The shock of being confronted with such a fundamental loss was devastating. I desperately wished that I could have taken back that request. Therefore, please use the following with caution.

Memory

Questions to Ask. Can the person recall recent events? Does the person frequently recall events and situations from the distant past? Is there a discrepancy between the person's account of his life and that given by others? What is the person's attitude toward his forgetfulness? Is there evidence of confabulation, filling in memory gaps with logical but inaccurate information? Does it occur spontaneously or only in response to questions? To sample short-term memory, ask the person to recall three objects immediately after seeing them and then five minutes after he has seen them.

Significance. The person whose immediate recall and short-term memory are impaired needs repeated instructions, reassurances, and reorientation. It is extremely difficult for him to learn new things. On the other hand, the person with well-preserved long-term memory can feel quite comfortable discussing events from the past. These long-ago memories can be a wonderful commodity to add to any interaction. Open-ended questions and insistence on facts by the caregiver may produce confabulation and should, therefore, be avoided. Remember that confabulation is the person's effort to give current events meaning. It is not lying.

Expressive Language

Questions to Ask. Does the person talk around a word without being able to get to the point (circumlocutions)? Does he sometimes use non-existent words (neologisms) or near-miss words (paraphasia) to express his thoughts? Is there a significant discrepancy between the person's output when he is speaking spontaneously and when he is replying to questions? The former is usually more fluent and expansive, while the latter may be sparse and labored. Is automatic speech, nursery rhymes, counting, etc., easier than conversational speech? Are emotional utterances preserved when formal speech is defective?

Significance. Caregivers will have to make more effort to listen for the message behind the words, pay more attention to nonverbal communications of the person and pay active attention to the context in which the message is delivered. They must avoid the temptation to dismiss garbled language as evidence that the person is "totally confused" or to correct the person who uses the wrong words. Also, caregivers should not assume intact language function on the basis of good automatic or spontaneous speech. For more detailed discussion of language and communication see Chapter 9.

Receptive Language

Questions to Ask. Even if the person's speech is totally impaired, it is still necessary to determine whether he can understand what is said to him. Can he point out a specific object when presented with a selection? Can he indicate a response to simple yes or no questions? Can he follow simple orders to do things such as picking up an object or clapping his hands?

Significance. If the person has difficulty here, caregivers will have to minimize dependence on verbal communication and augment their speech with nonverbal cues such as gestures or concrete objects. Also, they must not assume that the person whose speech is impaired is unable to understand what is being said.

Written Language

Questions to Ask. Can the person follow a simple written instruction, for example, "Clap your hands"?

Significance. Even though the person may be able to read aloud, he may not understand the meaning of what he reads. If not, reliance on written notices or signs for orientation or reminders should be discontinued.

Attention

Questions to Ask. Is the person's attention easily aroused and sustained? Does he concentrate or is he easily distracted? Can he attend to a simple task, such as reciting the months of the year backward? How many digits can he repeat forward and backward? Seven and five, respectively, are within normal range.

Significance. The person may have difficulty remaining with a task. He may wander from the topic during a conversation. He may not notice—and therefore not remember—occurrences. He is likely to need frequent reminders of the goal of his activity, and may need to be repeatedly redirected to the task. An environment free of distractions will be essential to this person's successful performance.

Abstraction

Questions to Ask. Can the person extract meaning from statements that do not reflect a concrete reality? Can he understand instructions that involve objects that are not immediately present? To sample, ask him to interpret a proverb such as, "Rome wasn't built in a day." Also ask him to explain the similarity between two different objects, such as a turnip and a cabbage (both vegetables), or a plane and a bicycle (both means of transportation).

Significance. A person with problems in this area will find it difficult to grasp explanations or conceive of future events or consequences. Instructions should be given, or questions asked, with concrete cues.

Judgment

Questions to Ask. Does the person's behavior suggest a change in his social judgment? Can he solve simple problems? Can he anticipate the consequences of an action? To sample, ask some situational questions, such as "What would you do if there were a fire in your house?"

Significance. This person may be prone to embarrassing faux pas. He will need direct and explicit one-step instructions in order to succeed. He will need help to resolve simple problems or mix-ups and avoid catastrophic reactions.

Insight

Questions to Ask. Is the person aware of a change in his abilities? Is his self-assessment realistic? To what does he attribute this change? How does he account for his move into care or day-program? How does he accept help? To sample, closely observe the person's reactions when offered help. Note how the person describes the facility and his relationship to it. Open a nonthreatening conversation about general changes one experiences during the course of a lifetime.

Significance. The person who lacks insight or has an unrealistic assessment of his own abilities will need additional supervision, as well as added support when confronted with difficulties. If the person seems so inclined, it may help to enlist a social worker or counselor to help initiate a discussion with him of the "memory problem."

Visuospatial Perception and Visuomotor Coordination

Questions to Ask. Does the person judge space and direction accurately? Does he seem to know where his body is in relation to objects in the environment? Does he know left and right? Does he lose his way easily? To sample, ask the person to copy a simple line drawing of a square, intersecting triangles, or a cube. Can he construct a square or triangle with sticks or matches?

Significance. The person with deficits in these functions will tend to be insecure and more dysfunctional unless provided with a consistent environment. He is likely to have difficulty learning his way around, and is liable to become lost. He will function better given simple, multisensory instructions.

Praxic Functions

Praxic functions involve the integration of the steps that constitute skilled and learned movements.

Questions to Ask. Can the person accurately carry out, on command, previously learned motor acts, such as making a fist or a ring with thumb and little finger? Can the person imitate such actions? Can he complete a complex task that consists of several steps, such as folding a letter, placing it in an envelope, and sealing the envelope? Does he have undue difficulty dressing, become muddled when inserting limbs into clothing or put garments on the wrong way around?

Significance. A person with deficits in these areas will require step-by-step cues and instructions to complete complex tasks. This person will do much better given simplified tasks that exploit familiar patterns. He is likely to become more flustered if the caregiver tries to direct him to do things that he does not understand or tries to explain to him how he has gone wrong when he makes a mistake.

5 | Functional Assessment

Functional assessment examines an individual's ability to manage tasks of daily living in the face of a physical, intellectual, or emotional disability. It is generally used to tell care providers and researchers which tasks the individual is able to complete independently, with which ones he requires assistance, and which will need to be done for him entirely. The results of functional assessment can be used for a variety of purposes. The choice of instruments or formats will depend on the purpose for which the results are to be used.

Some functional assessments are useful to evaluate the level of care that an individual requires in order to determine program placement, service, and reimbursement levels. Others add objective evidence to the process of deciding whether an individual should continue living alone or pursuing potentially dangerous activities such as driving. Such assessments are also used to track progress of the disease and to measure the effects of interventions and medications. Finally, functional assessment identifies the kind of help that an individual will need to maintain an optimum quality of life. Since this book focuses on the direct caring process, this chapter will address this last aspect of functional assessment.

Traditional assessment instruments consist of a list of personal and instrumental activities of daily living, either real or simulated, from the basics such as dressing, eating, toileting, and grooming to household management, transportation, handling medications, and more. Most of these assessments ask the examiner whether the person can perform the task and if so to what degree. Although this is very useful information, it is not sufficient for planning effective interventions. If a functional assessment is to help the caregiver identify the kind of assistance that the person needs to live comfortably, it must:

- be client-centered, that is, reflect the person's priorities and standards;
- describe the person's approach to a task in specific terms;

- determine the nature of the assistance that the person needs to complete the task adequately;
- identify those skills that remain in the very disabled person who is no longer able to complete any task; and
- be based on a conceptual model of function that is specific to the kind of impediments the person faces.

No one assessment format or instrument can fulfill all of these requirements. However, separate instruments address one or several of these perspectives. Three different instruments are discussed here, as a sampler, to illustrate the kind of thinking that is vital to the process of effective functional assessment.

The Functional Performance Measure

The Functional Performance Measure (Carswell et al. 1992) is a valid and reliable instrument that describes the individual's approach to a task, identifies the kind of intervention that the person needs to achieve, and is based on a conceptual model specific to dementia. It also credits the person with various levels of participation when completion of the entire task is no longer possible.

The Conceptual Model

A functional assessment instrument must be sensitive to the specific impediments or vulnerabilities created by the person's disability. For example, a cognitively intact person with a physical challenge will have little difficulty demonstrating the full extent of her ability to brush her teeth, even if asked to do so in a medical office. The environmental context will have little influence on the quality of her performance. The cognitively impaired person, on the other hand, will be heavily influenced by the relevance and familiarity of the surrounding in which she is asked to perform. The assessment format must take this into account.

The instrument must also direct the assessor's observations toward those performance features that are particularly jeopardized by the illness or condition in question. In other words, it must tap into those specific aspects of performance that are most likely to interfere with the person's ability to complete a given task.

These were the issues that the researchers had in mind when they set out to develop a model that would uniquely describe the cognitively impaired person's approach to any task. They asked the following:

- How does this person's approach to a task differ from the approach of a person who is not cognitively impaired?
- What elements are missing in this person's approach that are present in that of a person without cognitive impairment?
- What factors uniquely influence the performance of this person and would have little or no influence on the performance of a cognitively intact person?

To answer these questions, the investigators made videotapes of healthy individuals performing certain common tasks and of persons with Alzheimer's disease performing the same tasks. They presented these videos to a panel of eleven health professionals and family caregivers. The panel members were first given a training session in making consistent and objective observation. They were then asked to identify the elements that distinguished the performance of the cognitively intact persons from that of the persons with Alzheimer's disease. These elements were termed "subcomponent skills," and were sorted, coded, and categorized. The researchers then asked the following questions about each of these subcomponent skills:

- Is this skill essential to the successful completion of the task?
- Is the presence or absence of this skill observable by the assessor?
- Is this skill related to cognitive ability?
- Is this skill degraded by the process of a dementing illness?

Those items that met these criteria eventually formed categories of subcomponent skills that are fundamental to function, that are vulnerable to the disease process, that influence the performance of persons with Alzheimer's disease, and that are observable by the assessor.

The model suggests that functional performance comprises three interrelated elements: (1) the quality of performance demanded, (2) the environment within which the activity is performed, and (3) the person's behavior. Each of these three elements forms an axis in the model. Each represents an aspect of function that influences the person's performance and needs. All these elements, then, must be taken into consideration during the assessment process.

Quality of Performance

What quality of performance is acceptable? To take dressing as an example, we need to know the standard to which this particular person aspires. If we accept putting on a sweatsuit, perhaps even back-

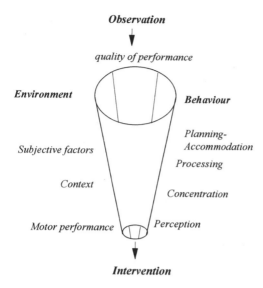

Conceptual model of the subcomponent skills for functional performance in activities of daily living for persons with Alzheimer's disease (Carswell et al. 1992)

wards, as adequate dressing, the person who can neither button nor cope with multiple or complex garments can, according to this assessment, dress independently. However, an orchestra conductor who is unable to tie a bow tie, according to this assessment, requires help in dressing. The standard to which the person needs to perform to maintain the quality of life that he and his caregiver desire determines how the other two axes are evaluated. It also influences the kind of support and attention that the person will need on the other two axes.

Environment

The environment axis identifies factors that are not directly related to cognitive ability but that have a significant impact on the performance of a cognitively impaired person. It is composed of three subcomponents: subjective factors, context, and motor performance. Subjective factors include the person's motivation, interest, and willingness to perform the task. Context refers to the physical environment—the familiarity of the place, the person's comfort in the environment, and the appropriateness of the place and time for the task. Context also refers to the person's familiarity with the task and to its gender/culture appropriateness for this particular person. Motor performance refers to the person's physical ability to perform the movements demanded by the task, and includes factors such as strength, range of motion, balance, and physical coordination.

The model holds, then, that any assessment task must be undertaken willingly by the person, in a familiar, appropriate and comfortable environment, and must be within the person's physical capacity to perform. A compromise in these factors will affect performance and must be noted, first, to account for the person's ability or inability to perform and, second, to identify those circumstances that are necessary for that individual's optimum performance.

Our maladroit orchestra conductor, for example, may be perfectly able to tie his bow tie in his own bedroom, when there is no pressure or distraction. Backstage, with the orchestra tuning up and only the music on his mind, he is all thumbs. If he needed only to put on a sweatsuit, perhaps even backwards, he would be fine. When it comes to bow-tying, however, he needs a quiet, distraction-free, and unpressured environment. If circumstances demand that he tie a bow backstage, someone must be available to help him. An effective functional assessment outlines exactly these circumstances for the caregiver of a cognitively impaired person.

Behavior

The behavior axis describes the direct efforts of the cognitively impaired person or describes specifically how he employs those subcomponent skills that are vulnerable to the disease process. These skills are the following: (1) perception; (2) concentration; (3) processing, which refers to the ability to initiate, sequence, and persist with an activity to its end; and (4) planning/accommodation, which refers to the ability to recognize and correct errors or accommodate change during the course of an activity (Carswell et al. 1995). Each of these four skills is further divided into subskills that more narrowly define those areas in which the person is competent and those with which he needs help.

The Process

The assessor's observation of the person's approach to a task, in terms of these subskills, forms a performance profile that determines where and how the person will need to be helped. The functional performance measure guides the assessor to ask questions such as:

- Does the person recognize the objects related to this task?
- Does the person maintain attention to the end of the step?
- Does the person recognize an error in his performance?
- Does the person initiate the task spontaneously?

In this way, the caregiver obtains an image not only of what the person is able or unable to do but also how he actually approaches the task and what is impeding his success. The caregiver might observe, for example, that the person is having difficulty dealing with certain decision points in an activity. This, then, is the area where intervention will be needed.

The Functional Performance Measure enables caregivers to derive effective methods of intervention. It forces them to look closely at the circumstances in which the person is being asked to perform. It also asks them to define the standards to which the person must perform in order to meet his needs and the needs of those around him, and in this respect is client-centered. It is a standardized test; its scores can be compared with previous scores to determine the progress of the disease or track responses to interventions and medications. It also supports the concept of a working partnership between the cognitively impaired person and the caregiver.

The Canadian Occupational Performance Measure

The Canadian Occupational Performance Measure (COPM) is an occupational therapy assessment instrument that goes a step beyond the partnership concept of care (Law et al. 1994). It is based on the principle of client-centered practice and responds directly to the person's priorities and perspective (Canadian Association of Occupational Therapists 1991). It is featured here because it raises some important issues about the relationship between the caregiver or provider and the client in dementia care.

The COPM measures a person's own assessment of her performance and her satisfaction with that performance in three areas of occupational performance: self-care, productivity, and leisure. It also invites the person to rate the relative importance of each problem or competency in conducting her life as she wishes. It is not an objective measure of functional ability, but rather a subjective evaluation of occupational performance. In other words, it describes the way a person is experiencing her life and her satisfaction with that experience. This is an important concept, because although functional ability supports occupational performance, it does not, as such, define it.

The COPM is a standardized way of asking the client the following:

■   What aspects of function connected with self-care, leisure, and productivity are most important to you?

- How would you rate the quality of your performance in each of these areas?
- How satisfied are you with the quality of your performance in each of these areas?

The administration of this instrument must be adapted to accommodate the person and her abilities without compromising its reliability and validity. A semistructured interview and formal rating and scoring process would not suit a person who has a pronounced cognitive impairment. However, depending on the person's insight and communication skills, information can be gathered in any number of ways, such as a conversational interview, an interview with the person's caregiver, or observation of nonverbal behaviors. Information can also be inferred from knowledge of the person's past preferences and habits, and gleaned from incidental encounters.

The use of the COPM ensures that the client's perspective is actively and formally taken into consideration during assessment and care planning so that the ensuing management plan really serves her interests. Here is an example:

Mrs. G. has Parkinson's disease and a moderate degree of dementia. She finds it very difficult to feed herself. Her motor coordination is poor. She often drops food onto her clothing and loses food from her mouth. Her attention span at the table is poor. Meals take a long time.

A plan based on objective assessment and aimed at maximizing Mrs. G.'s independence at the table provides for the following:

- adapted equipment, such as a padded spoon, a heated "scooper" dish, and a colorful apron to protect her clothing; and
- social intervention: positioning Mrs. G. in a quiet corner of the dining room to minimize distractions, and providing frequent reminders to continue eating.

Despite these interventions, meal-time performance did not improve; Mrs. G. continued to lose weight and started to show signs of depression.

Now the situation is described from a client-centered perspective.

Mrs. G. has some difficulty expressing herself orally because of dysarthria and cognitive impairment. Nonetheless, information gathered from conversations with Mrs. G. and her family, as well as from observations and incidental remarks, reveals that Mrs. G. has never been interested in either cooking or eating. All her life, she would rather grab a bite and get to the tennis court. What was important to her was being among people and being physically active. Her physical appearance and social decorum are also very important to her. She has always been a pragmatic woman.

When we put this information, along with additional insights and inferences, into a client-centered perspective, the following picture emerges.

On a scale of 1 to 10 in the COPM format, Mrs. G. would have rated herself as follows:

	Importance	Performance	Satisfaction
Self-care			
Eating	1	5	1
Appearance	8	2	2
Leisure			
Socialization	10	2	2
Exercise	8	2	2

The management plan that was in place focused on the area of least importance to Mrs. G. and compromised the areas that were most important to her. Furthermore, it limited her ability to use her most valued skill, her ability to socialize. Without this profile, no one would have thought to ask Mrs. G. whether she wanted someone to feed her. In the course of the conversation that this profile precipitated, however, this became an obvious alternative. Indeed, that was exactly what she wanted, but had never been able to insist upon. She had asked several times, but the staff interpreted these requests as "lack of motivation to be independent."

Considering this new perspective, another plan was developed. Mrs. G. was encouraged to sit at meals among her friends. An attendant was assigned to feed her. It was explained to Mrs. G.'s tablemates that the feeding was due to Mrs. G.'s physical disability, and no one minded. Because she was being fed, she did not soil her clothes and could dress nicely for dinner. She finished in time, and with plenty of energy left to attend social activities and exercise group, both of which were very important to her. Her mood improved and the weight loss stopped.

On reassessment with the COPM, Mrs. G. would likely have rated herself as follows:

	Importance	Performance	Satisfaction
Self-care			
Eating	1	2	8
Appearance	8	8	8

	Importance	Performance	Satisfaction
Leisure			
Socialization	10	10	10
Exercise	8	4	8

Mrs. G. was not formally evaluated with the COPM, but had she been the productivity aspect of her profile would probably have been as dismal as the self-care and leisure portions had been. One day, she came upon an attendant who was busily writing as she waited after work for her ride home. Mrs. G. asked her what she was writing so intently. The young woman said it was a list of all the things she had to do that evening when she got home. To which Mrs. G. answered, "What I wouldn't give to be so busy that I'd have to make a list."

When a person is no longer able to complete any of the tasks of daily living independently, the traditional functional assessment shows very little in the way of competencies. The person in care is, therefore, perceived as incompetent. This is why there is so little emphasis placed in long-term care on productivity. It is an attitude that isolates residents from a major human activity—work.

The kind of information that the COPM collects is important as it pertains to the life of the cognitively impaired person. It is equally as important with respect to the caregiver's needs. The caregiver is also a client in this situation and needs the same kind of consideration as the cognitively impaired person. The COPM is a valuable tool in formulating a plan that will ensure that the caregiver's needs, assets, and challenges are also properly addressed. The concept of care planning that considers the individual needs and abilities of caregivers, both family and paid, warrants serious attention. The COPM is a valuable step toward such care planning.

Assessment of Severely Impaired Persons

A cognitively impaired person retains certain abilities well into the very severe stages of the illness. A useful assessment should include some way of formally identifying those abilities in even very impaired persons. How often do we hear staff say, "Did you know that she can . . . ?" A program director tells of how her staff got through to a very impaired lady by using a remaining ability. A very dependent lady had been sitting with her eyes closed ever since she had arrived at the facility. Many people had tried to get her to open her eyes by telling her about all the wonderful things she would see. It was all to no avail. Then someone found out that this lady loved violin music and played her favorite piece for her. The lady recognized the music and opened her eyes. When such treasures are uncovered, it is wonderful. When they are not, it is a tragedy. That is why such discoveries should not be left to chance. Very few assessment instruments are sensitive enough to evaluate the retained abilities of very impaired persons. Such evaluation is important because it enables care providers to use those remaining skills to enhance communication and provide meaningful sensory and social stimulation.

The Severe Cognitive Impairment Profile is one such instrument (Peavy et al. 1996). It was designed specifically to evaluate the abilities of very impaired persons. It explores not only the person's competencies in attention, language, memory, motor ability, conceptualization, arithmetic, and visuospatial abilities, but also the individual's comportment, including cooperation and socially appropriate responses. It not only credits the person's correct responses, but also credits and, more importantly, describes the individual's effort. This is a formal way of recognizing the person as being able, for example, to respond to her name or to notice an object and try to use it, even if inappropriately. It credits the person who is able to sing a familiar song and also credits the person who makes any sound at all in an effort to sing. These are the tiny responses to which an individual sensory and social program can sometimes be affixed. Once a positive reaction is identified, a program can grow. For more details see the sections on activity programming and group work.

Is It Realistic?

Some will say that the general application of this approach to functional assessment is unrealistic, that the resources are not there to conduct such assessments on each program participant or resident. The real question is whether programs can afford not to invest their resources in such assessments. Trying to get people to do things that they are not able to do and not giving them the opportunity to do the things they can are far more costly in terms of staff time and energy. Furthermore, no price can be placed on the morale and spirit that are lost to frustration and burnout among both staff and participants when this kind of information is not available or not used.

When programming is based on a realistic appraisal of each individual's abilities, the pressure and feeling of defeat that unrealistic expectations and unreasonable standards create is removed. Both staff and program participants flourish. They express their competencies, rejoice in their successes, and, remarkably, often exceed expectations.

Preventing Challenging Behavior

If we look closely enough at many "challenging" behaviors, we can usually see in them the person's search for security, control, identity, affection, or a sense of purpose or achievement. The goal in prevention is not to stop the behavior but to address the needs that lie behind it. When we succeed in creating a situation that anticipates and therefore meets these needs before the person feels them, many of these challenging behaviors can be prevented.

This approach brings to mind a story of a clever waitress.

New on the job, this waitress was given the tables at the back of the restaurant. One of these tables was frequented each day by the establishment's grumpiest and stingiest customer, a rude man who seemed set on making life miserable for every waitress who served him and who, besides that, never tipped. His habit was to come to his regular table, order a vodka martini and a bowl of soup, drink his martini, and doze off. When he awoke, his soup would be cold. He would call the waitress and demand that she warm it for him. Then he would order another martini and a filet mignon. When the steak arrived, he always insisted that it was too rare and sent it back to the kitchen. He would finish his meal in a grumpy mood and go out, leaving nothing behind but a trail of ill will. The new woman had to cope with this scourge of waitresses. Instead of merely tolerating his behavior, she decided to do something about it.

When she saw him coming into the restaurant, she ordered the vodka martini on her way past the bar and had it waiting at his table. Just at the time he was waking from his nap, she passed by his table and offered to take his soup, saying, "That must be cold. Here, let me warm it up for you." It was just as easy to take the soup back to the kitchen then as later, perhaps even easier because it fit into her own pace. By the time she brought the steak and asked him if it was done well enough, the old man had mellowed so much that he grunted and said that, yes, it would be fine. "Are you sure?" she asked. "Yes," he nodded with a faint smile. "It is just fine." This gentleman became her best tipper. The clever waitress had succeeded in serving the gentleman's needs before he had to draw attention to them.

This is what we aim to do for the person with Alzheimer's disease. When we have achieved this happy state, outsiders look at our programs and marvel at what an easy job we have. "You people do nothing here but enjoy yourselves," they say. "You should come to our place and see what it is like to work with people who really have Alzheimer's disease." We smile at one another and say, "Thanks for the compliment. We'll keep working at it." That is exactly what it takes, a lot of hard, conscientious, and focused effort. When it works, when we see cognitively impaired persons interacting and achieving, when caregivers feel that they make a real contribution in the face of a devastating illness, we see that it is really worth it.

The preventive approach is based on the conviction that most problematic behavior is not a direct, linear consequence of cognitive impairment; it is the result of a lack of fit between the cognitively impaired individual's needs and the supports provided by his environment. Until a cure is found, there will not be much that we can do to change the person's needs and challenges. There is, however, much that we can do to change the environment.

Why Prevention?

Problematic behavior often indicates a lack of fit between the person's needs and the capacity of the environment to serve those needs. This creates a stressful situation. By the time behavior becomes problematic, things have usually been developing for some time. The person has been trying to cope with the challenge. His efforts have somehow brought him into conflict with the rules and needs of his care providers and coparticipants. It is then that we see that something is amiss and try to correct it. By then, however, it may be too late for the most humane and effective interventions. In addition, the person has already suffered. The stress has also threatened that person's trust in his environment. Trust is one of the most vital tools that we have in caring for cognitively impaired persons. Once trust and dignity are threatened or lost, the job of the caregiver becomes much more difficult.

Another reason for prevention is that not all people respond to stressful situations with behavior that we consider problematic. Those who suffer without drawing attention to themselves also need excellent care. The case of Mrs. X. is an example.

> Mrs. X. has always been concerned with hygiene and has had a little stress incontinence, but nothing that she has mentioned to anyone. In this new facility, where all the washrooms are discretely tucked out of sight, she cannot find the toilet. She is ambulatory. Incontinence is not a problem. No one is concerned about Mrs. X. She manages to come across a toilet once in a while and makes a point of going each time, just in case. Her day becomes a constant search for the toilet and she is plagued by the fear that someone may discover that she has had accidents. She is busy, albeit unproductively, much of the day. She gets in no one's way. Whereas Mrs. Y., who is regularly and openly incontinent, is the subject of much staff concern, is shown to the toilet regularly, and is reminded to go before most activities, Mrs. X.'s plight is unknown to the staff. She is suffering; her anxiety builds and her function declines. Unless someone identifies this as a problem, her needs will go unmet. Eventually staff start to find soiled underwear stuffed into odd places in her room. They ask her about it and Mrs. X. denies that the underwear is hers. She blames her roommate who has been "plotting against her." Now there is an obvious problem that must be "managed."

Another reason for prevention is that it is proactive rather than reactive. It is much more positive and, therefore, much more rewarding. An orientation toward prevention keeps caregivers actively looking at processes and practices to determine if they are ideal. It gives them an opportunity to challenge the old ways of doing things, and it gives them permission to make improvements. It gives them a mandate to be creative, and develop programs that grow and break new ground. All this makes the job fun.

When we can rectify or avoid stressful situations before they result in difficult behavior our programs and our relationships are generally more positive. The practical outcome is that staff who enjoy their work are more stable. They take fewer sick days, and are less inclined to leave. Families and caregivers of participants are pleased with the program and are more likely to recommend it to others. Things just work better.

Individual staff members and family caregivers at home who are able to maintain a preventive attitude are more resistant to burnout. Although it may take more effort and require greater alertness, prevention takes less emotional energy and affords the caregiver a much greater sense of control. Caregivers report that a sense of futility and lack of control in the face of a demanding situation are far more draining than simple hard work.

The Realities

It takes much more than the proverbial ounce of prevention to avoid a pound of cure. The adage fails to do justice to the amount of work that prevention really takes; it would be more accurate to say that a couple of pounds of prevention is worth two pounds of cure. Prevention requires effort and resources. Care providers, especially in the institutional sector, may not always believe that they can spare these resources. They usually feel that way because their resources are already stretched to the limit running after the problems that haven't been prevented.

It is really a matter of putting the investment of time, planning, and effort up front. This requires some faith in the process. Such faith is often difficult to muster because it is a common belief that behavior problems are part and parcel of dealing with persons who have Alzheimer's disease. This common belief suggests that problem behavior is inevitable and that the only way of coping is to respond with a management plan once the behavior appears. It is true that there is a challenge in caring for persons with cognitive impairment. It is a challenge that must be met with a two pronged approach: prevention and management.

Some Fundamental Questions

How Do We Perceive Behaviors?

Are behaviors our problems or are they the person's efforts? If we take our cues from the cognitively impaired person and start seeing behavior as that person's effort to cope and to communicate a need, then we cease seeing the behavior as something that must be eliminated. We start looking at alternatives and understanding instead of trying to impose controls.

How Do We See Our Role with Cognitively Impaired Persons?

The health care system has for a long time imposed a paternalistic relationship between care provider and care recipient. The social system has softened that perspective somewhat. The person with cognitive impairment needs to feel a partnership. This person is not unique in having that need; the difference is that she cannot cope with anything less.

Lacking insight, she does not accept the paternalistic relationship, and balks against it or withers under it. This person does not willingly accept care because she does not appreciate the need for it, and this challenges the caregiver to closely examine every interaction with this person.

How Do We Understand the Behavioral and Functional Manifestations of Dementia?

Our capacity to serve the interests of anyone with a disability is directly contingent on our understanding of that disability and its implications. Can you imagine planning an arts and crafts program for physically disabled persons without taking into account whether they have sufficient use of their limbs? That would be ridiculous. However, we often figuratively walk a cognitively impaired person right into a wall by asking him to do something that is impossible for him because we do not recognize his disability and its functional consequence. It is easy to do this because dementia is a hidden disability, but it is nonetheless real and pervasive.

How Do We Respond to the Individual's Needs?

The person with cognitive impairment is challenged in his capacity to meet basic physical and psychosocial needs. Unless we remain mindful of both of these types of needs, we may, despite all our good intentions and efforts, actually be frustrating the person. For example, if security is interpreted only as the need to keep the person physically safe, it may lead the caregiver to restrict movement and limit potentially dangerous activities. The consequences might be the person's loss of control and autonomy, diminished sensory stimulation, and fewer opportunities for meaningful and fulfilling occupation. The frustration of these needs then leads to other problems. The person continues to seek stimulation, occupation, and autonomy by engaging in what may be even more troubling behaviors. More restrictive "solutions" are then applied and more and more needs are frustrated. Unless the situation is addressed from the perspective of meeting personal needs, the cognitively impaired person and his caregivers become locked in a continuing spiral of frustration and restriction.

A preventive approach recognizes the cognitive losses that are most likely to impede a person's performance, helps the person compensate, and enables him to function in a way that best meets his needs. Some compensatory mechanisms become general policy in a facility or program. These are approaches and environmental features that would be likely to enhance the function and comfort of anyone, but are particularly helpful to the cognitively impaired person. An example is ensuring an adequate level of glare-free and shadow-free lighting. Other measures would be instituted as part of an individual's personal plan; examples would include calling the person by a particular name or title, offering specific activities, and providing assistance in a specific way that addresses the individual's special needs.

Identifying and Addressing Basic Needs

Security

Safety needs figure highly. A person who cannot make sense of his environment or who cannot retain information from one minute to the next is very vulnerable. His world seems very unpredictable. Much of the behavior we see can be traced to the person's effort to either flee or to defend himself and whatever is precious to him. Trusting relationships give the cognitively impaired person a refuge when things become difficult. A predictable and consistent environment with everything that he needs visible and clearly accessible contributes to his sense of safety. Security also means having the opportunity to express competence, industry, creativity, and other talents in a failure-free and accepting environment.

Affection

The need for affection and intimacy may lead a person whose judgment is impaired into socially embarrassing situations that may be stressful for the caregiver. Many behaviors that appear overtly sexual in nature are actually an effort to obtain simple human contact. It has been demonstrated in many programs that the deliberate offering of touch and nonsexual opportunities for the mutual expression of warmth and regard not only reduces the incidence of troubling behaviors but also enhances the quality of the behavior of residents toward one another and toward staff (Archibald 1994). The whole issue of sexuality among persons in care facilities and in those with dementia is, fortunately, in the process of critical review.

Inclusion

We derive our sense of belonging from fulfilling certain roles in our families, society or workplaces. The need to maintain his identity and significant function may keep a person going through the routines of a previous occupation. But poor judgment and planning may get him into trouble. Dementia can also isolate a person and make him feel like an outsider. A person who no longer feels important or valued may withdraw or lash out. He may fight for his integrity by covering up and denying errors, or by blaming others.

An orientation that identifies opportunities for meaningful activities as a major component of care can do much to alleviate these feelings. Meaningful employment is important both in the individual's home and in a facility or day program. It enables the person to continue being a valued contributor. People, even those with dementia, tend to live up to expectations. If the person feels like a useful, valued member of a community, his behavior will reflect that self-image. And the person who feels he is without value or purpose will behave accordingly as well.

Control

Much of the resistive and aggressive behavior we observe in persons with cognitive impairment is actually an expression of their need for control. Reports of incidents of "aggressive behavior" very often identify precipitating circumstances such as a caregiver removing clothes, giving medications, giving a bath, changing underwear, relocating the person. This raises the question of who is perpetrating the aggression. What is the person actually doing but defending himself and fighting for control?

Control over one's body, possessions, and immediate space is a very powerful need, and is very easily threatened but just as easily satisfied. Try the following exercise with a friend. Hand your friend a glass of water and ask her to let you drink from the glass. Sit on your hands and allow yourself to experience a total loss of control as someone else decides how much water reaches your lips, how fast you must drink, and whether it is important that your clothes stay dry. Remember that feeling.

Now ask for another drink. This time, place one finger anywhere on the hand of the person as she holds the glass of water. You exert only a little control, but it makes a world of difference. You can direct the flow of water. You can orient the glass. You are involved, not a passive object. Now translate the significance of this experience to other activities, such as personal care.

Any involvement or active participation that we can afford the dependent person has a huge effect on her sense of control, and must not be overlooked. So ask her to hold the soap. Give her the washcloth. Ask her to raise her foot, or give you her hand, or look in the mirror and approve of the job that you are doing on her hair.

Accommodating the Losses Most Commonly Associated with Alzheimer's Disease

The following is a review of compensatory approaches to the cognitive deficits described in Chapter 2. Few of these approaches would be offensive to the cognitively intact person. If they were incorporated into our everyday life, many would make life easier for anyone with whom we come into contact. However, for a cognitively impaired person, most of them mean the difference between security and apprehension, efficacy and failure. Taken as a whole, they can make a profound difference in such a person's behavior.

These approaches must become as much a part of a cognitively impaired person's daily experience and must be taken as seriously by care providers as medications and biomedical interventions. This is fundamental to excellent dementia care. A cognitively impaired person's experience of the environment and her interaction with the people in it has as much impact on her system as do medications and diet. No one would think of substituting some other medication for a diabetic's insulin. It would be a real problem if every staff member in a facility were not aware of a diabetic resident's dietary restrictions. The staff member who sees a diabetic patient in distress or unconscious due to excessively low blood sugar is compelled to give that person whatever she needs, no matter how much time it takes. Comments such as "That is just glucose-seeking behavior," or "I don't have any glucose on me right now, but, here, this aspirin I have in my pocket should do," or "She will just have to wait until I have time or I will never get my job done" are unthinkable in the context of biomedical interventions. They are no more acceptable in the psychosocial context.

Coping with Memory Problems

Chapter 2 reviewed the behavioral and functional consequences of memory loss. By enlisting the following principles in our interactions with cognitively impaired persons, we can do much to lessen the impact of the disability and prevent the resultant behaviors.

- Stop relying on recent memory.
- Provide consistency.
- Avoid open-ended questions.
- Use and accommodate to long-term memory.

Many of our moment-to-moment operations rely on short-term memory. This is the kind of memory that is most quickly lost in Alzheimer's disease. Because we rely so heavily on short-term memory for our daily functions, we unconsciously also expect a cognitively impaired person to remember instructions, reminders, and things that have just happened. Open-ended questions, expectations that the person will remember instructions, and, especially, admonitions for not having remembered, are especially unwise. Probably worst of all are statements such as "I just told you that" or "I just gave it to you; what did you do with it?" They roll off the tongue so easily, in a moment of exasperation, that we are hardly aware of them. To a cognitively impaired person such statements can feel like stinging arrows. They create apprehension and mistrust, and diminish the person's self-esteem. Taking care to avoid such comments will help to forestall many problems. Instead of asking the person about events in the recent past, inform the person about them and then ask his opinion. Open-ended questions about recent events invite confabulation and all of its attendant problems.

Consistency is a memory-impaired person's lifeline. If a piece of information is repeated consistently enough, it eventually becomes ingrained and will persist. The process by which this happens is called *procedural memory* and is discussed in more detail in Chapter 7. The power of consistency and repetition is confirmed by the success of programs that maintain a consistent and predictable routine. This is not to say that schedules are important, but rather that routines, the general flow of one event after another, the way activities are introduced and set up, the words that are used to announce an event are. When program participants are given the cues which help them anticipate coming events, and the time to prepare for them, they are much better able to maintain their sense of control and security. Many challenging behaviors, such as pacing, clinging, defensiveness that comes across as aggression, and efforts to leave the premises are due to anxiety and fear of the unknown. A comfortably predictable and, hence, secure environment contributes significantly to the prevention or substantial reduction of these behaviors. This is an important factor to consider when facility administrators must decide between rotating or stable staffing patterns.

Long-term memory usually persists well into the disease. Therefore, we should exploit the person's memories from the more distant past. The pleasure of remembering and a sense of success are possible when programs take advantage of old memories. Encouraging the person to talk about the past, share their accumulated wisdom, or recite familiar poetry are all ways in which caregivers can take advantage of this retained ability. There was a time when talk of the past was considered to be an unhealthy regression. How can talking about the things that the person understands the best and enjoys the most be anything but healthy and promote anything but healthy behavior? What better way to contribute to an individual's sense of competence, control, and efficacy than to give him the opportunity to talk about something he knows really well.

A person with memory loss is far more likely to be familiar with household items that date from her younger years than with the modern versions we now have in many facilities. Telephones, bathroom and kitchen fixtures, and paper towel dispensers have all changed a great deal in the past twenty years. Single-handled faucet fixtures and touch-tone phones may mean nothing to this person. Articles that cognitively impaired persons are expected to use in program or residential areas should be of a style that they are likely to recognize. Imagine the feelings of insecurity and incompetence you would have if you were surrounded by things that you did not know how to use.

Supporting Language

Many difficult behaviors come from the cognitively impaired person's frustration at the misunderstandings and isolation that result from lack of communication. The process of establishing and maintaining positive communication is discussed in detail in Chapter 9. Some fundamental principles are:

- Learn the person's vocabulary: words and expressions that he uses and those he is most likely to understand.
- Do not correct his vocabulary or insist he use the right words.
- Attend to nonverbal language.
- When speaking, keep things simple, but don't condescend.
- Support words with gestures and props.

The first and most important adjustment a caregiver must make with respect to language and communication is to assume full and unilateral responsibility for understanding and being understood. The second is to realize that this is not the time to try to improve language; it is the time to communicate. Therefore, instead of correcting the person's errors or trying to encourage him to learn the correct word or name, the caregiver should learn the person's vocabulary. If the person persistently says "Mary" when referring to his wife, Alice, make a note of it. Let other care providers know. Then when he says "Mary," you need only confirm your understanding that he wants to talk about his wife. This approach avoids introducing a negative distraction into the conversation and lets the conversation proceed smoothly.

It is also very useful to identify certain important words that the person is most likely to understand and to let other care providers know what they are. One gentleman with severe aphasia had been admitted to the hospital for tests. The nursing staff had a great deal of difficulty making him understand that he was not to leave the floor. Among the words that his wife left for the staff was the word "impractical." This was a word that he understood to mean not permitted or, simply, not to be done. Using this word helped to resolve much of the frustration associated with this gentleman's care. Whenever staff found him on the way off the floor, or doing anything else he was not supposed to do, they told him that it was "impractical" and, understanding what was said to him, he calmly stopped. Although it did not help him remember that he was to stay on the ward, it did make it easier for the staff to redirect him in a positive manner each time he tried to leave. Such lists of words and common errors are important enough to be placed on the person's chart in a long-term care facility or on a personal information sheet in the home, for in-home care providers.

Caregivers must also be aware of, and note for others, tendencies that the person might have, such as swearing or rambling. Recording these is especially important for newcomers so that they do not attribute such tendencies to poor manners, take offense, or, worse still, reprimand the person.

Communication consists of far more than words. Tone of voice, inflection, facial expressions, and gestures all add to and clarify verbal language. When listening to what a person is saying, be attentive to nonverbal messages as well; these often convey meaning more accurately than words. One lady whose language had been severely disrupted by a stroke was able to say nothing but profanity. The staff had to rely exclusively on her tone of voice and occasional gestures to interpret her intentions as informative, gentle, funny, complaining, or caring. They learned to respond to her as though she had actually said, "Good morning. How are you?" or "My hip hurts," instead of the stream of curses that she was actually uttering. It is unlikely that many people with Alzheimer's disease will experience such an acute problem, but the need for caregivers to be attentive to nonverbal language is always important.

While paying attention to the person's nonverbal language, caregivers must also be aware of their own. Body language can either contradict or support what is being said. Be very careful that there is no contradiction between these messages. Use nonverbal messages not only to support your words but also to elaborate upon and clarify them. Support what you say with commonly used gestures. When speaking about an object, point to it. Avoid figures of speech that might confound a person who has difficulty coping with abstractions. Keep the conversation concrete. If there seems to be any doubt, confirm that the person has understood your meaning correctly.

Promoting Attention

Behaviors such as failing to stay with an activity, disrupting group activities, wandering, restlessness at meals, crying out, and irritability are the result of an inability to focus attention and withstand distractions. The following interventions and management techniques will do much to limit and prevent such behaviors:

- Reduce distractions.
- Provide meaningful and consistent cues.
- Give information in small, manageable parcels.
- Reorient the person as necessary.
- Adjust expectations to the person's observed abilities.

The healthy person's attentional system has the capacity to filter out extraneous and insignificant stimuli. It does this so efficiently that caregivers are often not aware of the noise, movement, and other distractions that are going on in the areas where cognitively impaired persons are trying to work, play, or otherwise function. The biggest offenders are radios and televisions, public address systems, conversations held by caregivers over the heads of residents or program participants, and service traffic going through program areas.

All of this irrelevant activity can make it impossible for a cognitively impaired person to function at all. Imagine trying to study for an exam in a room with fifty people who are watching the last game of the World Series. Would you be a little irritable? Televisions and radios left on as background music or entertainment have no place in a general program area for cognitively impaired persons. This kind of noise also distracts the staff from their primary role, interaction with the residents. The strongest support to a cognitively impaired person's attention is the undivided and focused attention of the caregiver. Staff should learn to respect the importance of their own attention, as well as that of their coworkers. They must not interrupt each other or allow themselves to be interrupted when engaged with a cognitively impaired person.

The television should be in a small room away from the general activities area. Anyone who can follow the intricacies of soap operas and talk shows will also be able to find the television without difficulty and will, furthermore, enjoy the program without interruption. Anyone who cannot find the television will probably not be able to follow the programs either.

There are programs and videotapes that even very impaired persons can enjoy. These should be put on and the people gathered to watch them. When the program or tape is over, the television should be put away. Music should be treated the same way. Radio with commercials, talk, and unpredictable music is usually meaningless and distracting for most persons with moderate to severe cognitive impairment. It is far better to put on a tape of music or songs that either a group or an individual will enjoy. Individuals can listen to music through headsets.

Whereas the noise from radios and televisions is distracting, the life-size pictures on big-screen television can add to the disorientation and misperceptions of persons who are already vulnerable. Family members and visitors sometimes wonder where the tales of mayhem and misdoing in the nursing home are coming from. One need only look at the nightly news to have a fair idea.

Everyone working with a cognitively impaired person must know how to give orienting and supportive information in small, pertinent, and manageable parcels. Too often the caregiver's effort to orient or re-direct a person's attention actually proves to be even more distracting. This can precipitate problematic behavior, such as irritability and wandering. Consider the following well-intentioned effort of a caregiver to keep a disoriented person in touch. "Good morning, Mr. Smith. I am Sally, your nurse for today. I am here with your breakfast, fluffy pancakes that will give you plenty of energy to enjoy this sunny day in July." Information must come to such a person on a need-to-know basis in small bits that he can process. What does Mr. Smith really need to know right now? The identity of the person coming toward him with a plate? What is on the plate? The weather? What month it is? How much of this can he figure out for himself? Does he recognize pancakes when he sees them? Mr. Smith can handle only one or perhaps two bits of information at a time. He is likely, then, to have grasped very little of what has just been said to him. He may actually feel overwhelmed and no better oriented than he was to begin with. He may even be so unsettled by this encounter that he gets up and leaves his breakfast uneaten. A better approach might have been simply, "Good morning, Mr. Smith. Here's your breakfast."

In another example, a well-intentioned caregiver sits with a cognitively impaired person during his meal and repeatedly coaxes him to eat. Each time the person is distracted or loses touch with the task at hand, she explains to him why he should eat, what they will do as soon as he is finished and how the food will be spoiled if he lets it get cold. In doing this, she is actually, albeit inadvertently, distracting him and increasing the load on his attentional system. The redirection cues she uses should be determined by this person's needs and abilities. It may be that simply touching his shoulder or hand will be enough to redirect him to the task. This kind of prompt consumes very little of his attention, yet successfully helps him to refocus on the meal.

Many of the challenging behaviors seen in persons with Alzheimer's disease are a consequence of excessive demands and unrealistic expectations. Inattention, agitation, and restlessness are often due to anxiety created by the pressure of these expectations and demands. If caregivers insist that a person must participate in activities that exceed his attention span, they are actually exacerbating the problem. The expectations of caregivers should be adjusted to a person's observed abilities. When this is done, remarkable things usually happen. The person relaxes; his function may improve, and he may even exceed expectations. The aim of care is to offer a person opportunities to express competencies, not to enforce compliance with a caregiver's inflexible expectations.

> One gentleman would not sit at the table for more than a few minutes at a time. Staff members ran themselves ragged trying to get him back to the table. He was losing weight. When the staff relaxed and offered him foods that he could pick up and carry away, they also removed the pressure that was feeding his restlessness. To everyone's amazement, he gradually started to stay longer at the table. They also discovered that much of his restlessness was due to the fact that he could not handle the full-course meal that was customarily served. He could manage sandwiches and other finger foods much more easily. When the staff simplified his place setting and offered him meals that could be eaten with only one utensil, this better suited his abilities and his restlessness diminished markedly.

Dealing with Poor Judgment and Insight

Lapses in the cognitively impaired person's judgment also contribute to problematic behaviors. Much of this can be prevented by the caregiver's foresight. The most troubling behaviors, however, develop when the person is forced to justify, correct, or account for errors that result from her faulty judgment. Some approaches that can be used to prevent these problems are:

- Anticipate potential errors.
- Avoid putting the person on the spot.
- Limit choices.
- Preserve the person's trust.
- Don't argue or try to convince.
- Back away at the first sign of antagonism.
- Enlist the person's retained capacity for logic.

Preparation is the best prevention, and the errors we anticipate are the least likely to happen. This is especially true when we are dealing with a person who is not likely to look beyond the immediate situation, who is not likely to check labels, and who is likely to take things very literally. When asking a cognitively impaired person to do a task, make sure that she cannot make a mistake, or that whatever mistake she does make will not have any serious consequences. Remember that the purpose of asking the person to do things is to give her the pleasure of doing. It may take longer to failure-proof a task than to actually do it yourself, but that is the decision that a caregiver must make. One family complained that their mother had spoiled the dinner after their counselor had advised them to let her do the dishes. They served dinner on dishes that their mother had washed with lemon oil instead of dish liquid. No one had thought to check under the sink to see what could be mistaken for dish detergent.

Decisions and choices require abstract thinking, which is often impossible for a person with impaired cognition. Therefore, limit choices to those that will give the person pleasure, not anguish. Limit the choice to alternatives that will all be equally desirable. For example, if Mother enjoys choosing what she wears, let her choose from several outfits that are equally appropriate. If, on the other hand, it is essential that you leave to go to the doctor's office, do not ask her if she is ready to go. Simply inform her that it is time.

Because a person with limited ability for abstraction is likely to take your words literally, avoid using figures of speech when giving instructions or directions. Use demonstrations and concrete objects to illustrate what you mean. Also be prepared for the person to do exactly as she is told, no more and probably no less.

Most caregivers can deal with instrumental problems, no matter how exasperating or time- and energy-consuming they are. What is truly painful, though, is the behavior of a person who feels threatened, needs to justify or defend herself against what she perceives as unfounded accusations. This happens when a cognitively impaired person's errors are brought to her attention and she feels she must account for or correct them. Although few of us would intentionally put another individual into such a situation, there are times when expressions such as "Why did you . . . ?," "Couldn't you see that . . . ?," and "Why didn't you . . . ?" just seem to come out by themselves. These outbursts are the product of a caregiver's exasperation, but have the effect of putting the cognitively impaired person on the spot. Remember that the person tends to take your words literally. She is not likely to understand the rhetorical nature of the question and will feel compelled to give an accounting. This can spawn defensiveness, which can lead to accusations and arguments that no one will win. As soon as this kind of confrontational question slips out, the caregiver should check the person's reaction. If there is none, let it drop. If the person is prepared to answer, however, let her know that you realize she had a good reason and that it is okay. This reaction will help to calm the situation and will preserve the person's trust.

A person who has impaired judgment is also likely to have difficulty controlling her emotional expression. This means that her reactions to situations such as the above may be much more extreme than one would expect from a healthy individual. With this in mind, the caregiver should pull back at the first sign of the person's upset and simply let her emotions run their course. Nothing is gained from exhorting the person to control herself; it will only make matters worse.

The last item on the list at the beginning of this section, enlisting the person's retained capacity for logic, is likely to surprise many readers, because the inability to think logically is frequently cited as one of the symptoms of Alzheimer's disease. Many cognitively impaired persons, however, retain the ability to see the logical connection between two points. What they usually lack is accurate information to connect. It is often possible to help a cognitively impaired person see your perspective if you begin with a point to which she can relate, and then lead her, step by step, along the logical path to your conclusion. There is, of course, no guarantee that she will either agree with your reasoning or remember whether she agreed or not a moment later, but this approach does help you explain why you see things a certain way, in a manner that respects her intelligence and preserves your relationship. This issue is treated in more detail in Chapter 7.

Helping Techniques That Support Perception

Many difficult behaviors stem from the person's sense of vulnerability, insecurity, apprehension, and anxiety. Anyone who puts himself, for a moment, in the shoes of a person experiencing the perceptual limitations caused by dementia will readily understand why a person with cognitive impairment is prone to these feelings much of the time. The person's effort to cope with an environment that is distracting, ambiguous, or misleading places such a load on his system that he has little left with which to handle other challenges. His responses are likely to be elopement, searching and pacing, combativeness, or learned helplessness. Caregivers should therefore provide as lucid an environment as possible by taking the following measures:

- Eliminate distracting, ambiguous, or meaningless stimuli.
- Provide multisensory orientation cues.
- Maintain a consistent environment.
- Use colors and textures to create meaningful contrast.
- Provide high-level, full-spectrum lighting.
- Eliminate glare and shadows.

Wandering, combativeness, withdrawal, and other perplexing behaviors can arise from the person's misinterpretation of environmental cues and the anxiety that such misinterpretations create. Public address announcements become part of conversations. Glare distorts space and the contour of objects in front of it. Shadows may look like solid objects. It sometimes takes a critical eye to identify those stimuli that might be distracting or misleading to a cognitively impaired person because our systems simply ignore such things. For example, we would not see flowers on a carpet as anything but a design, while a cognitively impaired person may be so afraid of tripping over them that he refuses to venture into the room. Caregivers must acquire the habit of appraising the environment objectively. Is the furniture in the room obvious by its shape and color? Large bold prints on upholstery can obscure the shape of a sofa and make it difficult for the person to figure out where to sit. The navy used "Razzle Dazzle" camouflage, which consisted of large colorful patches on their transports and battleships, in World War II. Even though the enemy could see a ship, they could not tell what kind of ship it was because its contours and fittings were disguised by the design.

We do not want our residents or participants to experience the same disorientation.

Caregivers should also note whether the furniture in the room is distinct from its background. If furniture is not clearly visible against the background of the carpet and walls, the person may trip over or bump into it. Are the paths for moving about obvious in the room? A person who cannot see a clear path to his destination will not feel comfortable moving about. Are the walls and floors clearly distinct from one another so that the person can easily discern the limits of the room?

These considerations are just as valid for small spaces as they are for large ones. The place setting at the dinner table, for example, should be free from clutter and have obvious limits. Table implements and food should be distinct from their backgrounds and clearly recognizable.

All the environmental cues the person receives in a place should be consistent with the activity that occurs in that place. If a dining room, for example, really sounds, smells, looks, and feels like a dining room, the person's attention to dining and his ability to eat will be enhanced. If, however, the room sounds like a fish market, smells like a craft room, looks like a bingo hall, and feels like a train station, what does a person do?

A person with dementia is also likely to be experiencing the sensory changes of old age. Poor hearing, especially of high tones, clouding of the cornea that distorts colors and makes glare intolerable, and the inability to cope with abrupt changes in lighting add to the load already on the cognitively impaired person's perceptual system. Therefore, noise control and consistent, high-level lighting that is free of shadow and glare are essentials in a dementia care program.

It is best if the environment, both at home and in a facility or day program, stays the same. In the home, caregivers should try to keep things as the person is used to them. We often see a decline in function and an exacerbation of behaviors provoked by anxiety and insecurity when things in the home change. In a facility or day program area things should stay consistent so that participants and residents have the opportunity to become accustomed to them. If there is a change, such as seasonal decorations, it should be confined to a certain, accustomed area and should not alter the general layout.

Techniques to Help Motor Organization

Apraxia, the inability to organize one's movements to perform a familiar task, can make a person seem recalcitrant or uncooperative.

Efforts to convince or pressure the person to act may evoke anger and frustration. The caregiver must realize that if the person could perform the act she probably would. Therefore, reasoning is not the issue, organizing the movements is. Here are some techniques to help a person with motor organization problems get started and work through a task or operation:

- Place the person in a context that will automatically trigger an appropriate pattern of actions.
- If the person becomes stuck or loses track of the activity, let it go and start over from the point where the person seemed to know what she was doing.
- Start the activity and then let the person's natural inclination take over.
- Anticipate and help with decision points.
- Avoid trying to convince a person to do something that she cannot do.

The automatic patterns that we rely on to complete most routine tasks are triggered by environmental cues. We are often not even aware of the actual trigger. If someone hands us an object, our hand simply reaches out and grasps it. This is the mechanism we try to engage for the cognitively impaired person with apraxia. Instead of telling her to pick up the pencil, simply hand it to her. Hold out the coat that you want her to put on, hand her the ball of yarn that you started to wind and ask her to continue. Make sure, however, that the automatic pattern that you are trying to elicit is available. If the lady already has something in her hand, she will not be able to reach for the pencil. In that case you may have to tell her to put it down or, better still, put out your hand as a cue for her to give it to you.

A daughter described the following episode that she had observed between her parents, Charlie and Alice.

> Charlie came in from the yard and took off his hat. Alice told him to take off his coat and come into the kitchen for tea. Charlie just stood there holding his hat. Alice called him into the kitchen. He came in still wearing his coat and holding his hat. Alice noticed what was wrong; Charlie couldn't take off his coat while he was holding his hat. She told him to put down his hat. Charlie reached up to his head and said that he had no hat on. "The hat in your hand," said Alice. Charlie glanced down at his hand, but had forgotten what he was supposed to do with the hat, and just said, "Oh, this hat," and continued standing there. When Alice reached out her hand and told her

husband to give her the hat, however, she triggered a familiar pattern. Charlie handed over his hat, took off his coat, hung it up in the hall, and came into the kitchen for tea.

Sometimes the cue that will trigger a desired pattern of movement is obvious. Sometime it is a little more obscure. A homemaker wanted to involve a client in familiar chores such as vacuuming, but was having difficulty getting her to participate. She had been bringing her own vacuum cleaner from home because the client's old one was too cumbersome. One day she failed to bring her own and was about to start using the client's old machine, when the client came over, took the vacuum cleaner wand from her hand, and said, "Here, you have to know how to handle this thing, dearie. You're doing it all wrong. I'll take over here." The modern machine was just not familiar enough to trigger the habitual pattern.

Sometimes triggers just appear. It is an observant caregiver who can pick them up and use them. One very impaired gentleman did nothing in the day program but wander about restlessly. Staff knew that he had been an avid card player, but could not get him involved in any game. A volunteer was sitting with him one day, just handling a deck of cards, when the gentleman said, "Hit me." The volunteer recognized this as a cardplayer's term for "Deal me a card" and dealt him one. "Hit me again," said the man, and the volunteer dealt him another card. Then the volunteer handed the gentleman the deck and said, "Hit me." He was dealt a card. So began what became a regular game of dealing cards, something that this very impaired gentleman could do and consistently enjoy.

Some complex, multiple-step tasks will have to be broken down into individual steps, with each step treated as a separate task. While dressing, for example, the caregiver may need to hand over each item of clothing, one at a time. The complex operation of putting on a series of items can be overwhelming and create resistance and anxiety.

By all means, avoid trying to convince the person to do something or explaining how it should be done. One of the most dramatic and overwhelming behavioral patterns displayed by persons with Alzheimer's disease is the *catastrophic reaction*. This can happen to anyone when the system is overloaded. For example, you overslept and are late for work. You spill coffee on a clean shirt. The babysitter calls to say she will be late. The cats get into the garbage. When, on top of it all, the phone rings, you break down and give a blast to the poor woman who just dialed a wrong number. This is precisely the mechanism that is at work in a cognitively impaired person. The provocation, however, may not always be so obvious to us. The person has been asked to do something. She wants to do it but does not know how to start. Someone is talking to her while she is trying to concentrate. She makes a move and the caregiver says, "No, not that way." She stops to think and the person keeps talking. Then he moves her in a direction that she doesn't understand. She is trying so hard and he is just getting in the way. She loses control and hits him. Such outbursts can usually be prevented, but it requires a keen sensitivity to the person's subtle reactions during the course of an interaction. In most cases, the person is telegraphing her feelings long before the outburst occurs. Too often the caregiver is so intent on getting the job done that he does not notice her discomfort.

Areas of Intervention

In the preceding section we looked at preventive measures from the perspective of accommodating various areas of cognitive deficit. This section looks at how the four basic elements of care—interpersonal contacts, environment, routines, and special activities—can contribute to preventing problematic behaviors.

Interpersonal Contacts

Every time two people pass or exchange glances, whether they realize it or not they are sending a message to each other. Because the cognitively impaired person is so dependent on her environment, each encounter has a significant impact on how she feels, and that, of course, influences how she behaves. Each caregiver, then, has many opportunities during the day to influence, either negatively or positively, the behavior patterns of the cognitively impaired persons he or she is caring for. It is everyone's responsibility to make sure that each of these encounters is as positive as possible. This happens when everyone

- shapes everything that he does and says to build and preserve the person's trust and sense of mastery,
- searches for and understands the capacities that still remain in each resident,
- looks for the meaning and purpose behind their behavior, and
- works to develop and sustain a partnership with them.

The cognitively impaired person's trust is the single most important asset a caregiver has. It is, however, easily lost. Unfortunately, many of the daily occurrences in long-term care undermine trust. Fortunately, few of them are necessary and most of them are easily eliminated. The following are just a small sampling:

- saying that things are okay when they are not;
- moving people who are in wheelchairs without warning and before receiving their permission;
- calling people by pet names;
- interrupting people at mealtime to give medication;
- entering people's personal space before receiving permission;
- removing plates, cups, or glasses before receiving permission; and
- presenting plates, cups, or glasses without warning.

Every caregiver should make a habit of asking, "Would I trust someone who had just done or said this to me?"

A sense of mastery is one of the most important things that a caregiver can offer a cognitively impaired person. All of the things that undermine trust also undermine the person's sense of mastery. When trust and mastery are gone, the person is left alone and vulnerable. This is when she resists dressing, bathing, and medication. This is when she accuses or cries that she wants to go home.

Even the most severely impaired person retains the capacity to experience emotions such as love, fear, sorrow, shame, joy, pride, and sympathy. This is why it is important to ask the person to please lift her feet when we want to clean under them, and why it is important to thank her after she has done so. A very impaired person's awareness of the environment must never be discounted, nor must her capacity to be sociable and to respond to social situations. Many overlearned patterns of behavior and automatic skills can still be enlisted to help a cognitively impaired person feel productive. The need to communicate remains even if the capacity to produce or understand words is lost. Therefore one must never overlook seemingly trivial means by which a cognitively impaired person can participate in any activity. When there is only a little bit left, everything that remains takes on enormous importance. Remember, a little bit is infinitely more than nothing. For more details about accommodating persons with very limited abilities, see Chapter 7.

Every encounter is an opportunity to strengthen the relationship. If the caregiver takes control, stops the vicious cycle of reactivity, and looks

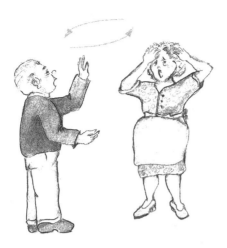

When behavior escalates, it is often because two people are caught in a cycle of action and reaction.

for a way to let the person feel well respected and supported, even a potential altercation can be such an opportunity. The challenge is to come out of the situation with both people feeling good. This is a win-win style of problem management. When disputes are treated in a win-win fashion, challenges posed by the illness do not go away, but problems due to mistrust, fear, and helplessness are prevented.

Here is an example.

Anne, a caregiver, is helping residents seat themselves in the dining room when she notices Mrs. K. in Mrs. L.'s place. She approaches Mrs. K. and asks her to move, but Mrs. K. is intransigent, insisting that she is in the right seat. This would not be a problem if Mrs. L. were not coming into the room and heading for the same chair. Anne sees a problem brewing and must think of a win-win approach. Instead of trying to convince Mrs. K. of her error she says, "Mrs. K., I know you really prefer this chair. However, could you do me a favor for just this one time, and sit in this chair over here. I would really appreciate it." This acknowledges Mrs. K.'s preference and invites her to be of service, something that most persons in long-term care seldom have the opportunity of doing. If Mrs. K. remains resolute, Anne will approach Mrs. L., take her aside as she comes into the dining room, and ask her to please do her a favor. The favor is to let Mrs. K. enjoy that seat just for this meal. She will let Mrs. L. know how much her concession is appreciated and thank her.

Environmental Adjustments

The Physical Environment

When we come into a place, we can generally tell by its style, layout, and atmosphere what we can expect, how we should behave, whether or not we belong there, and whether we will get all that we need there. If the place looks like an institution, it tells us that there are important people in charge. Unless we are used to being one of those in charge, we come here to do business, or to have things done either for us or to us. Many nursing homes have among their residents someone who is used to being in charge of such a place and continues to act as though he or she still is. However, that is not the case with most people. People do not usually live in institutional buildings. If we come to visit, we usually leave before dinner. If we eat, we usually have to pay. It is small wonder, then, that many cognitively impaired persons assume a passive role in institutions, persist in trying to get on with business or leave, and worry about meals and paying for them. In a home, on the other hand, even someone else's home, one comes as an equal. One might stay for a meal and never consider paying. Here one would just stay and visit, offer to lend a hand, and even lie down for a little rest.

Consider two different program environments. In one, the Day Away Program was housed in a chronic care hospital. Despite every effort to make it homelike, there was still the institutional main entrance, the elevator, and long corridors with the terrazzo floors and high ceilings of an institutional facility. Participants came happily because they enjoyed the program, but they came to participate as they would in a community center or other place where activities were arranged for them. They tended to wait for direction, and they were ready to leave when the activity was over. By contrast, in Charlottetown, Prince Edward Island, the local Alzheimer Day Program is housed in an old home. It has a country kitchen, wooden floors, a parlor with cove ceilings, a bow window full of flowers, a garden, and a toolshed. It looks like a home. Participants come in through the kitchen like old friends. They sit at the table and serve one another coffee. They lend a hand with the dishes, work in the garden, putter in the shed, prepare some lunch, and share a meal. Then they retire to the parlor, chat a bit, or just sit and visit. Someone may even have a little nap or go upstairs to stretch out on the day bed for a while. Although the atmosphere in both programs is very positive, each is a product of its own environment. The programming in each must accommodate the messages that its participants receive from their surroundings.

Much difficult behavior, as we have seen, is actually a search for security, identity, control, and meaningful occupation. The physical environment can do much to prevent difficult behavior by

- ensuring security, emotional as well as physical;
- accurately reflecting the individual's identity and promoting self-esteem; and
- offering opportunities for meaningful occupation and independence.

The following are some examples in which environmental features create either security or anxiety, and, therefore, either promote or prevent problematic behavior.

Nursing staff are the most important source of security and solace for most persons in long-term care. Yet nursing stations separate residents from these important people. Is it any wonder, then, that so many residents huddle at the counter and are reluctant to leave when the area becomes too congested? When nursing stations are eliminated, staff initially find it difficult to work without the structured space, but soon learn to work at a small desk with residents alongside or even at a kitchen table. Charts and medications need to be locked away; staff do not.

Staff meeting rooms are another place into which these important people disappear at every shift change. This sudden loss of security is probably a significant contributor to the phenomenon called "sundowning" (a tendency to become restless and agitated toward the end of the day, frequently observed among persons with dementia). When the walls are removed from the meeting room, residents are able to keep nursing staff in sight and do not have to interrupt every two minutes for assurance. As a result, staff conferences proceed much more smoothly. The Sneider Children's Hospital in Tel Aviv instituted a similar assurance measure for parents. Because the doctors were seldom visible on the wards, parents wondered if the children were really getting their attention. When they saw the doctors meeting and writing notes in the glassed-in conference rooms, however, they were assured that the full team was taking care of their children.

Earlier in this chapter we discussed ways of ensuring that the physical environment makes sense to the person with perceptual deficits. Such practices guard both physical and emotional security, which are in jeopardy when the environment encourages dangerous behavior such as exit-seeking, handling dangerous objects or materials, and exploring unsafe terrain. Even if an impaired person's access to these things is barred by locked doors, fences, or railings, the desire to explore, escape, or be occupied can cause the person to challenge the barriers. This can lead to frustration and even injury. There are some practitioners who would argue that camouflage is misleading and "unreal." However, judiciously used, it can save much grief. One facility painted a bookcase on the wall that contained a fire exit. In one stroke they decorated a bare wall and hid an enticing door without making it inaccessible. Another way to keep people away from a dangerous area is to make it obvious why they should not go there. This was done in one facility by planting raspberry canes on a fence that barred a dangerous ravine. There had been a problem with several gentlemen climbing the eight-foot fence just to see what was so special that it needed to be protected by an eight-foot fence. The raspberry canes were a natural barrier.

When something is removed, something else must be provided. Therefore, when access to something dangerous is denied, access to something safe and equally interesting must be offered. The space must provide interest points and promote satisfying activity. Walking areas must induce not only walking but stopping as well. They must offer a place to go, a place to rest or do something else before moving on. A sitting area with plants, fish, a magazine rack, and a window entices the person to come and spend some time. Tables and chairs invite people to socialize naturally. Even if they do not exchange a word they are still sitting together. If they are sitting side by side against a wall, each of them is sitting alone. The environment should also direct people's energy and attention to satisfying activity. Digging gardens, lawns for raking, carpet sweepers and brooms for cleaning the floors, and clotheslines are some examples. This aspect of the environment is discussed further in Chapter 10.

Some physical layouts can actually contribute to altercations and combative behavior. Dead-end corridors, especially those ending in locked doors, can create traffic flows that raise anxiety levels. Restless residents are attracted by the door and go down the hall, only to find the door locked. They become irritated and, in this irritated state, turn to see more restless people coming toward them. Someone bumps, someone pushes, someone may even be carrying a chair. Nerves are already on edge, and scuffles break out about one-third of the way down the hall. Narrow doorways through which there is a lot of two-way traffic, such as doors to dining rooms, create a similar situation. The problem with the hall is remedied by creating a sitting area out of one of the rooms at the end of the hall and making it a destination where the walkers can relax before heading back. Common rooms that have a lot of traffic should have two doors, large archways, or no walls at all.

Privacy is a powerful need that is often difficult to accommodate in a long-term care facility. This is especially true with a mixed population, in which some residents may not understand and, therefore, respect the personal space of others. Private rooms are usually available only to those who can pay for them. More and more, however, residences that accommodate persons with Alzheimer's disease are making private rooms available on the basis of need. On the other hand, shared accommodations are sometimes desirable. Roommates benefit from the stimulation and security of each other's company. When this is the case, or when private accommodations are not available, individual privacy and private space must still be available. A room set-up that does not compel one person to pass through the space of another can avoid antagonism and prevent disputes. Bookshelves and room dividers can contribute to privacy in a shared room. Private access to one's own window also enhances the sense of personal space.

The physical environment must also accommodate coexisting disabilities. The cognitively impaired person is less able to cope with other disabilities that may limit his autonomy. For example, the person with impaired mobility and balance will require secure handholds. Because of Alzheimer's disease, the person is less likely to choose handholds judiciously. He may persist in using unsafe towel racks and toilet paper holders instead of handrails. Only safe handholds should, therefore, be available. A person who has had a stroke may not be able to use one side of his body comfortably. His attention to things on that side may also be impaired. This person will need a customized environment to ensure that his disability is accommodated. The furniture, for example, should be oriented so that anyone entering his room approaches the person's good side whether he is in bed or in a chair. Handholds must be within sight and reach from his good side. Sometimes caregivers are so focused on one of the person's problems that they fail to see how the interplay of multiple problems is contributing to negative reactions and frustration.

Some environmental features may spark memories or associations for individual residents and so create difficult behavioral situations. One gentleman frequently came to the nursing station, at first requesting his money and then irately demanding it. The nursing station looked very much like a bank teller's window to him, and he became very angry when the staff told him that he had no money there. A commonly cited feature that brings back terrifying memories for Holocaust survivors is the tiled shower room. Although these are individual examples, they are the kinds of issues that should be considered in general environmental planning.

The environment must also respond to identity needs. It must reflect the person's being as he wants to have it reflected. Most people do not want their environment to reflect them as incompetent, childish, or dependent. For example, what does the traditional orientation board that announces the day, date, month, weather, next meal, and next holiday actually say about the people who live in a place? An orientation board announces to anyone coming in that the people who live in the place are unaware of the day, date, time, weather, and so on, and unable to find out for themselves. How useful is it to persons with cognitive impairment? Would it not be more useful to have large windows out of which the residents could see the weather if they wanted to know about it? Or a bank calendar to tell them the day, date, and month in a context that most people over sixty will recognize? How about a clock with hands on the wall to tell them the time? The smells of the place should tell them if another meal is on the way. General conversation and activity in the place should herald any holiday that is important for people to know about.

Large posted activity schedules send the same message as the orientation boards. They do not orient residents to the activities from which they can choose. They advertise to staff and visitors that the people who live in this facility need to be entertained and stimulated, and that the staff who work here do so only at specific times of the day.

Craft room displays also project a certain image of the residents, and the program staff must make sure that the image is appropriate. Potato prints done on construction paper and tacked up on a corkboard trimmed with crepe paper flowers are more suggestive of kindergarten than of a home for elders. The issue of making craft projects age appropriate for even very impaired persons is discussed further in Chapter 11. Whatever image of the person the environment projects is the image that staff, volunteers and visitors will internalize. Eventually, that is also the image that the person himself will receive. Either he will rebel against it with aggressive, combative, or resistive behavior, or he will succumb to it with childish and dependent behavior. Neither permits the person to truly be himself.

The Culture of the Environment

When people live and work together, they do so according to an established framework of values, beliefs, and standards. Their culture is

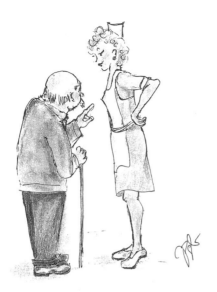

"Young lady, I have fought in two world wars, survived three wives, managed five hockey teams, and hired and fired more people than I can count; and *you* are telling *me* it's time to go to bed!"

expressed in actual practice; it determines people's relative status, which in turn determines the direction in which information, responsibility and influence flow. It also determines the priorities and norms by which achievement is evaluated and the consequences of anyone's failure to conform. Everyone, including a cognitively impaired person, thrives in an environment that accommodates the individual skills, needs, and limitations of all its members; where information, responsibility, and influence are openly shared; where the failure of an individual to meet the norms represents either a need in the individual or a need to reevaluate the norm, and not a fault; and where, although each person might have a different role, every individual is openly recognized as being equally important and worthy of respect.

Adjustments to Routine

The daily routine of life in a long-term care facility usually represents a radical change from what most people are used to. Baths must be scheduled to accommodate many bathers. Meals must be served at set hours. Bedtimes and hours of rising accommodate shift schedules. Although some people can adjust, these changes create anxiety and resistance in some, and unsettle others to the point that they cannot cope. Readjusting priorities so that life can take on a more normal pattern, especially for those residents who cannot handle the radical changes, can do much to prevent difficult and resistant behaviors. The time and effort invested in making the change usually pay off in time saved arguing and coping with resistance, and in enhanced staff and resident morale. Chapter 13 describes the experience of a nursing home in which the morning routine was adjusted to accommodate each resident's habitual and most comfortable pattern.

Much difficult behavior is also prevented with a flexible and tolerant approach. Everyone needs a break from routine. Who has not fallen asleep fully dressed in front of the TV? Who has not eaten so much popcorn during a movie that he didn't want supper, but was too hungry to go to bed without a snack? Everyone also has up days and down days. Sometimes an impaired person requires only to know that he has a say in the matter.

Specialized Programs and Activities

Many difficult behaviors are simply the result of having nothing to do. As long as activity programming remains the responsibility of a few specialists, this will continue to be a problem. When, however, everyone involved with a person feels a responsibility for how that person spends his day, many of the problems dissolve. A person need not be active during the entire day. There must be time for contemplation, observation, and just simply being. The program plan must, however, be satisfying to each individual; this requires individual planning with clearly stated objectives. The plan must also be reviewed regularly to ensure that it continues to meet the person's needs, abilities and interests.

Is It Realistic?

Professional caregivers who feel the pressure of numbers and schedules are likely to throw up their hands when offered this challenge, and say, "We do not have the time to do things this way. We cannot spend fifteen minutes distracting a gentleman away from the door. As much as we would like to, we do not have the time to find that old alarm clock, watch him tinker with it, or chase around after all the pieces he's tucked away heaven knows where. We have to bathe so many people in such a short time that we cannot spend a half hour with one person letting her just enjoy the experience."

Lack of time is a chimera that has no place in dementia care and is often the result of misaligned priorities. Experience actually shows it. Whenever a gap in the bathing schedule permits the luxury of a leisurely bath with that resident who really needs it, staff remark that that person's day, and consequently their own, just seems to go better. The reality is that the cognitively impaired person forces us to spend the time one way or another. Either we invest the time and effort up front by addressing his or her needs for security, control, efficacy, inclusion and affection, or we spend the time undoing, redirecting, and otherwise dealing with the consequences of frustrated needs. Life with a cognitively impaired person is usually a combination of both of the above. Everyone benefits if it is more weighted toward the former. This shift seems difficult, especially when the tradition in health care is so deeply rooted in efficient, standardized, instrumental care, but it is by far the best way to go.

No one of the approaches discussed in this chapter is a "silver bullet" that will, on its own, prevent difficult behaviors. Each technique or approach is part of a management or interaction philosophy that must be applied as a whole. It must also be applied critically. In every interaction, the caregiver must be aware of the cognitively impaired person's challenges and needs. He must also be alert to the person's reactions and know how this encounter is affecting her. The approaches, especially the interpersonal contacts, do not come about spontaneously out of good will. Care providers need to be taught these approaches. They need opportunities to practice and they must receive consistent feedback about how they are doing. They also need the chance to voice their concerns and questions when they see things that are not working. It is the responsibility of supervisory staff to give that training and feedback as part of their ongoing supervisory and teaching roles. If the practice is left to the good will and insight of individuals, application is inconsistent and residents get incongruous messages. This is when behavioral problems most often emerge.

| 7 | Using Well That Which Remains:
But I Thought You Said He Can't
Remember? |

This chapter, about using the cognitively impaired person's retained abilities, naturally follows and is an extension of the topic pursued in the previous chapter. By promoting the cognitively impaired person's retained abilities and eliciting the expression of his true personality, we can help prevent many of the behaviors that caregivers find so challenging. Much of this behavior comes from the person's effort to apply retained abilities to current problems or to continue deriving pleasure or satisfaction from activities for which he has some abilities but now lacks others. For example, the gentleman who removes all the light fixtures in the facility retains his manual dexterity and enjoys being busy but now lacks the judgment to apply his skill appropriately. Our challenge is to recognize his dexterity and industry as worthy attributes and to direct them toward a pursuit where they can serve everyone well.

Another factor contributing so commonly to problematic behaviors is the failure of the program to acknowledge or account for the person's true nature and personality. A lifetime, perhaps eighty to ninety years of experience, have gone into creating this individual. This needs to be not only acknowledged but celebrated. It is another precious commodity that must not be squandered.

Retained Abilities

Even in the face of severe deficits, most persons with dementia can

- remember things from the distant past;
- hold an opinion and offer advice;
- perform habitual, overlearned patterns of behavior;
- learn new habits;
- enjoy pleasurable sensory stimuli;
- respond to and express emotions; and
- follow a logical train of thought.

It would be absurd not to acknowledge and make full use of the abilities that the person retains. Just as every individual is unique in the degree and nature of disability the disease process inflicts, every person is also unique in terms of the degree and nature of the abilities that are spared. Sometimes the retained skills are obvious. Sometimes we have to dig for them. Some of them might come as a surprise. It is always a delight to find a treasure when one believed that all was lost.

Old Memories

If they are given the recognition they deserve, old memories can be absolute jewels for both the person with Alzheimer's disease and the caregivers (Sheridan 1991). Having memories of things the way they used to be means that this person knows things. Perhaps she even knows things that her caregiver does not and could learn. Recognition of this competence retrieves for the cognitively impaired person the position of sage and holder of wisdom and tradition that used to be part of the elder's role. We formalized this concept into a program in which the staff of a local small museum brought in artifacts, dating from about the turn of the century, to a group of cognitively impaired residents of a home for the aged. The purpose was not to tell the participants about the article, but rather to ask them about it. On a number of occasions the residents succeeded in clearing up some of the staff's misinformation about the artifacts (Zgola and Coulter 1988).

Old knowledge can also be used as a hook on which to hang new learning. The following example was discussed at the Fourth National Alzheimer's Disease Education Conference (Case study 1995).

> Mrs. C. had been very close to her son. While she was resident in an Alzheimer's disease unit, he passed away. The director and the staff agreed that she should be told. She understood the news and wanted to attend the wake. It was arranged and she wore her good black dress. In the days following the funeral, Mrs. C. continued to ask after her son. Each time the director explained about her son's death, it struck her as a new revelation and she experienced the pain as though it were the first time she was being told. The staff did not want to engage in any deception but did not want to continue exposing her to this anguish. One of them recalled the black dress that she had worn and that she recognized. The next time Mrs. C. asked about her son, the staff member showed her the dress. It helped her remember the wake. They left the dress out as a reminder. Although she continued to speak of her son frequently and did mourn his loss, she stopped asking about him.

This example underscores the importance of identifying those precious abilities that can help a person compensate for a disability. The initial choice had been between total competence and total incompetence. It meant either expecting Mrs. C. to cope with the information independently, which she obviously could not do, or avoiding the information altogether by telling a lie. That would have been demeaning. As it happened, the staff identified an ability that they could enlist to help her handle the information effectively.

Holding an Opinion and Giving Advice

Holding an opinion and giving advice are skills that come from a lifetime of experience. Every person, no matter how demented, has had a lifetime of experience. Dementia can only interfere with the verbal skills needed to share advice and opinions. But those can be overcome by alternative communications. Everyone knows the gesture that means "What do you think of this?" Everyone also knows the gestures that mean "Not so good" or "Splendid."

Another wonderful thing about opinions and advice is that they are never wrong. Although the person may be wrong about the facts of a matter, no one can say that her opinion is wrong. She may not be able to identify vanilla or vinegar by their smells, but she will certainly be able to tell you which she prefers. The only time that advice becomes wrong is when it is taken, not when it is given. The best thing, perhaps, about advice and opinions is that asking for them is probably the nicest gift one can give a cognitively impaired person.

Habitual Skills

In earlier chapters we discussed the automatic patterns of movement that we acquire during our lives. They come from having repeated an activity or a task so often that our body is able to carry on without our conscious attention. These are the skills that the old adage "like riding a bicycle" refers to. They are things that we seem never to forget. The cognitively impaired person does not forget them either. In fact, the person with Alzheimer's disease often relies on these old habitual patterns to get through the day. As long as circumstances fit, he can manage. As soon as circumstances change, such as with the death of a spouse, or a move to a new home, the old patterns no longer work and the functions that relied on them fall apart. The old patterns are still there, however. If we can create the circumstances in which they can once again be useful, we can let the person recapture the pleasure of comfortable achievement.

Sometimes the entire skill is preserved. Sometimes only fragments endure. It is like the person who plays the piano. At first, he is able to play a variety of pieces on request. Gradually his repertoire decreases, until eventually he plays only one or two themes over and over again. At every stage, it is up to the caregiver to find some gratifying way to apply whatever skill remains. The act of extending a hand in greeting to a person usually prompts an automatic response, a handshake. Even the very impaired individual is likely to respond appropriately to this gesture. When speech and conversation are no longer possible, such a gesture affords the person an opportunity to participate in an important social ritual.

Finding an outlet for the use of retained habitual skills is done by applying the process of activity grading (see Chapter 11 for an illustration). This process involves breaking an activity down into its individual steps and then determining which of these steps the person is able to do. Sometimes an individual is able to do the entire project. Sometimes he can handle only one simple repetitive step that contributes to its completion. This principle is the basis of Henry Ford's assembly line.

Some activities consist of only one or two repetitive steps. Sweeping, raking, folding linens, sanding wood, and stuffing envelopes are a few examples. There is a certain comfort in doing a repetitive task at which one is really good. The rhythm of the movement is soothing. The repetitive activity leaves the mind free to ponder other things or just drift. Giving a person with Alzheimer's disease such a task can actually be offering real comfort. It is a way of preventing behaviors that could become challenging. It is also a way of using the person's tendency to perseverate, that is, to get stuck in one step of a task, to the good. Instead of getting in the way of productivity, it can be used to benefit both the person and the caregiver. See the definition of perseveration in the section on attention deficits in Chapter 2.

Unfortunately, some very important habitual skills do not get the recognition they deserve, and as a result we may fail to give the person enough opportunities to express them. The ability to be polite in polite company is one. The ability to reach out to someone in need is another. These are abilities that persist long into any illness. They are so easy to access. They are also the abilities upon which much of our self-esteem hinges. Yet dependent persons are usually not given nearly enough opportunities to use them.

New Learning

That new learning can occur might come as a surprise to readers who have heard so often that a person with Alzheimer's disease does not acquire new information easily. True, it is not easy, and it takes time. However, under the right circumstances the person does learn. This is a very important insight for two reasons: (1) this ability is a valuable resource that should be used to enhance the life of the cognitively impaired person and her caregivers; and (2) the person does learn, whether we are actively involved or not. Unless caregivers understand the process by which the cognitively impaired person learns, they will not be aware of the kind of lessons that the person is learning during the course of each day. They will not know whether these lessons are ones that promote trust and security or ones that lead to isolation and mistrust.

The process by which the cognitively impaired person can learn, despite severe impairment of short-term memory, is called *procedural memory*. This is the mechanism by which we acquire habits and learn skills that we eventually do automatically. If something is repeated exactly the same way often enough, it gradually insinuates itself into our pattern of living. We might even forget having learned it. It is just there. It is a habit. This is the process by which most of us learned to tie our shoes. Someone showed us one way of doing it, over and over again, until it became our way of tying shoes. Had a different person showed us a different way each time, few of us would now be tying shoes easily.

Procedural learning relies on consistent repetition. It is one of the elements that contributes to the success of programs such as Day Away (Zgola 1987) and the Tea Group described in Chapter 12. Participants eventually learn what to expect. When they learn to expect pleasant, comfortable things, their apprehension, defensiveness, and anxiety disappear. They feel free to try things, to extend themselves, to really participate. The program works. The process by which caregivers can teach and the process by which the cognitively impaired person learns both operate on the same principle. However, each needs to be examined separately.

How Caregivers Can Teach

When a caregiver learns to use this process actively, he can actually teach the person new ways of coping.

One gentleman in the day program used to become restless each day in the early afternoon. The staff agreed that walking calmed him. They decided that one of them would invite him for a walk each day at about two o'clock. Because they could not ensure that it would always be the same person, they agreed that, for consistency's sake, they would all use the same phrase when approaching him. This phrase was, "Mr. A., you seem a little tense. Let's go outside and walk a bit." Mr. A. could understand this and happily went out. Each day he was in the program, the same thing happened. His afternoon restlessness ceased being a problem. However, the intervention had even farther reaching effects. One morning, Mr. A. approached a staff member, tapped her on the arm and said, "I seem a little tense. Let's go outside and walk a bit." The program bus driver later confirmed that Mr. A. had not wanted to leave the house that morning and that he had been quite nervous on the bus. Mr. A. had learned a new way of dealing with his tension.

This process also offers an exciting prospect for teaching persons in the early to middle stages of the illness new functional skills. There are formal teaching systems that are used to help patients with primary short-term memory loss called *surrogate memory*. The following, however, describes a less formal, yet still very effective, process.

Mrs. S. lived alone in a seniors' apartment. She had a regular homemaker. Her doctor's office was a short walk from her house. So was her hairdresser. Her friends in the building regularly took her to play cards and to weekly events at the local seniors' club. Her daughter worked nearby, called every day, and stopped in after work several times a week. Mrs. S. had everyone she needed close at hand, and she was driving them all crazy. She was calling them all many times a day at all hours of the day and night, asking when her next appointment was, when they were coming to visit, when they were going to take her out. While everyone around Mrs. S. was upset, Mrs. S. herself was frantic. Her apartment walls were covered with yellow sticky notes with cryptic messages, names, telephone numbers, times, and dates— none of them complete or making any sense to her. So she was calling everyone, desperately trying to keep things together. Each time she called and was given a piece of information, she wrote whatever bit of it she remembered on another sticky note and tacked it up on the wall.

The occupational therapist who came to see her first enlisted Mrs. S. as a partner to deal with the problem. They agreed that these yellow papers were not working. Some other, more effective, method of handling information had to be established. They did an assessment of Mrs. S.'s abilities. She was able to read an agenda calendar. She could find a given date and time. She could both read with understanding and write an item at the appropriate place. Furthermore, she agreed that such an agenda would be useful and went with the OT to buy one. She chose one that displayed an entire week at a time. They labeled this agenda "my book."

Then they agreed to remove all the yellow papers from the walls. This proved to be very difficult for Mrs. S. because she associated them very strongly with security. With much reassurance and repeated explanation as to how they were going to use "my book" instead, the yellow papers came down. The information on each one that they agreed could be useful was transcribed into the book.

Next, with Mrs. S.'s permission, the OT telephoned all the people whom Mrs. S. called regularly. She also had a meeting with Mrs. S.'s friends in the building. She explained something about memory loss and how it affected Mrs. S. She told them how the book was going to work and how they could help Mrs. S. learn to use it. Each time Mrs. S. called one of them, instead of giving her the information, they would tell her to look in her book. If she found the correct date and time, they would confirm it with her and encourage her. If she was unable to find it, they would tell her which date to look up, ask her to confirm it, and then praise her for her effort.

To increase the number of learning opportunities, the OT made appointments each day for Mrs. S. to phone her office at a given time and to expect a phone call from her at a given time. If Mrs. S. failed to call, the OT would call, remind her to look in the book, and confirm the appointment she had there. When the OT made her appointed telephone call, she asked Mrs. S. whether she had been expecting the call based on information in the book. Whenever Mrs. S. went to an appointment, the return appointment would be noted in her book and drawn to her attention. The homemaker also noted the time of her next visit, as did Mrs. S.'s friends and daughter. Everyone tried her best to be consistent.

At first, things were difficult. Each week, the OT visited and would have to explain how they were using the book and why. She would also find yellow papers back up on the wall. Mrs. S. remembered having quit smoking. It became a standing joke that breaking the sticky note habit was harder than quitting smoking. Mrs. S. sometimes became frustrated when people did not give her a direct answer over the phone. Several times she slammed the phone down in fury. Everyone needed support and encouragement at this point. Gradually, though, things started to settle down. The phone calls became less frequent. When Mrs. S. did call, she accepted the reminder about the book more agreeably. She started to use the book as a diary, even expanding on its use. Next to the reminder about a bingo game, she wrote, "Won." Next to the homemaker's appointment she wrote, "Get her to defrost the fridge." Then she wrote, "She did." As the book became more and more a part of Mrs. S.'s life, she started objecting to other people writing in it. She insisted on keeping all the notes in her own handwriting.

The book did not solve all Mrs. S.'s problems, but it did permit her to stay in the community for an additional two years. She died in the hospital after having had several strokes in quick succession. She never moved into a care facility. The intervention had come at a time when Mrs. S.'s family and friends were at the limit of their tolerance and could see no alternative to placement. The book left behind something very important too. The seniors in Mrs. S.'s building, the hairdresser, the staff at the doctor's office, and the homemaker had learned something that would affect the way they dealt with other cognitively impaired persons whom they encountered. They had also approached this problem as a team. That, in itself, had been a valuable experience.

If there is one rule that can be applied consistently in dementia care, it is that there are no rules that can be applied universally. One must always be prepared for surprises. People with Alzheimer's disease are not supposed to learn. They are not supposed to acquire new habits. Yet they do. Nancy Ewald, former activities coordinator for Manor Care Summer Trace, used line dancing in her exercise program. Her troop of line dancers, which included a number of cognitively impaired members, became so accomplished and developed such a stage presence that she took them touring as a traveling road show.

Mrs. F. had always hated rice—never even had it in the house. Her family told this to the live-in homemaker. The homemaker was Latin American, though, and rice was a staple in her diet. Mrs. F. was soon enjoying rice, too.

How the Person with Cognitive Impairment Learns

Procedural memory is also the process by which the person continues to learn from experience. This learning goes on whether we are aware of it or not. Lessons come from the small, consistently occurring incidents of everyday life. If these incidents are affirming, if they promote mastery, security, confidence, trust, and pleasure, this is what the person learns to expect. If, however, these small incidents defeat, shame, or frighten the person or tell him that he is dependent and incompetent or simply does not matter, then those are the lessons he learns. These opportunities for learning happen on their own. No one has to plan, sanction, finance, or realize them. They happen whenever

- someone moves a person in a wheelchair,
- someone notices a person heading for an exit,

- someone removes a plate from in front of a person,
- someone disagrees with a person, and
- on countless other occasions.

Think about each of the following examples and imagine what lesson you might eventually learn if the event were to happen to you often enough. Think also how the event could have unfolded otherwise to give you an entirely different lesson.

- You are walking down the hall and notice a door. There are lots of people coming and going through that door. You wonder what is going on, so you go and have a look. Suddenly someone takes you by the arm and tells you that you are not to go there. "There must be something very special behind that door," you think, "and I had better take a good look at it next time I have the chance." Or, you think, "If all those people are coming and going through that door, why can't I?" They must be holding you prisoner here. Now you must escape.

- You are sitting quietly, watching a conversation between your tablemates, when someone calls your name, approaches you, and says, "Excuse me." She waits for you to look up and asks you, please, would you mind if she moved your chair so that she can get by. You take a while to figure out what she wants; she said "please," so it must be important. Besides, she is waiting. So you say, "Sure." But you are not really sure what she wants. She then confirms to you that she is going to move your chair now. "Oh, move the chair," you think. "Okay," you say and brace yourself. The chair moves. She steps by. The chair moves back again. She taps you on the hand, gives you a smile and says, "Thanks." "That was easy," you think. You got a "please" and a "thanks" and what did you have to do for it? You didn't even have to lift a finger.

- You are walking down the hall and notice a door. You experience a certain sense of urgency that you can't quite pinpoint. It must be that you are supposed to go there for some reason or leave this place for some reason. You go for the door, but someone catches you by the arm and tells you that you are not to go there. You turn back reluctantly. Your sense of urgency grows.

- You had finished dinner and were just enjoying the last bit of coffee when you dozed off. You wake up and look to see if that last sip is still there just as someone's hand whisks the cup away. "That was *my* coffee," you think to yourself. "I didn't tell anyone that I was done with it." Or, "Have I just disappeared?"

- Your purse is gone. You know that man down the hall took it.

You find one of the nurses and tell her about it. She is really concerned about your purse because she is a woman and knows how important a purse is. She also says that she knows you are a reasonable person who would want to exhaust all other possibilities before accusing someone. Even though you know he did it, you'll give her that concession. After all, you are a reasonable person. You even agree to exhaust all possibilities, even some ridiculous ones, just to make sure before you go and get your purse from him. The purse turns up under the cushion of the sitting room sofa. The nurse tells you that she might have put her purse there too, if she had been at a sing-along and didn't want to leave such an important thing lying on the floor. If she can admit to doing such a silly thing, maybe you can too.

   ■   You are walking down the hall and notice that door, the one that, for some reason, makes you uneasy. You have to go and see what it is. You reach for the handle and start to open it when someone calls your name. You look around. She is coming toward you, smiling. She says your name again and says, "Please wait for me. I'm coming too." You wait. "Do you want to see what the weather is like?" she asks. That sounds like a good idea. You look out with her. It is a nice day. "Let's go for a walk right after breakfast," she suggests. She smiles at you again. As she holds the door and guides you back in, she says, "But let's get some coffee first." That also sounds like a good idea. You go back in.

It is true that the precipitating events simply happen. The caregivers' reactions, however, determine the impact that these events have on the cognitively impaired person. That impact determines what the cognitively impaired person learns about the place he is in and the people around him. We want to make sure that that learning is as positive as possible.

It has been suggested that this is actually stimulus/response conditioning, the kind of learning that is used in strict behavior modification programs and aversion therapy. I believe that this is a dangerous line of reasoning because it can lead to practices that are divisive and destructive to the relationship. Using the door as an example, a caregiver applying the behavior modification style of reasoning might conclude that, if the consequences of going to the door are pleasant to the person, he might be induced to approach the door more often. If, on the other hand, the act of going to the door is punished or otherwise made unpleasant, the person would be less likely to repeat it and would stay away from the door. Experience indicates otherwise. It shows that pleasant consequences do not induce repetition of undesirable behaviors, they induce relaxation, trust, and security and therefore a reduction in the anxiety and stress that lead to undesirable behaviors. On the other hand, unpleasant consequences such as punishment or admonitions simply associate the situation with distress and urgency and induce a flight-or-fight reaction. Therefore, if a pleasant incident occurs each time the person approaches the door, he may open it out of curiosity or try to leave just because it is there. But he is just as inclined to pass by. On the other hand, if an unpleasant incident occurs each time he approaches that door, he learns to associate the door with anxiety and distress. The normal response to feeling anxious and distressed in a place is to seek the closest exit, the door. It could be that much of the persistent elopement behavior that so troubles caregivers has actually been learned on the premises.

Sensory Pleasures

Alzheimer's disease interferes with a person's ability to interpret and understand sensations. It does not affect the ability to enjoy them. Unfortunately, as the person ceases being able to do things for himself, move about and interact with others, the range of his sensory experiences shrinks. He suffers from sensory deprivation. This is a serious condition, no less serious than starvation or dehydration. The human nervous system needs to be stimulated.

Smell, touch, taste, and the appreciation of melody and rhythm need no interpretation to provide pleasure. This is the time to let the person experience sensations that go beyond those offered in sensory stimulation groups, such as smells that come from little bottles or the textures on little plastic coasters. This is more than ever the time to be exposed to the aromas of coffee, burnt toast, onions frying, bread baking, and stew simmering. Any facility, no matter how institutional in nature, can have a coffeemaker, toaster, waffle iron, crock-pot, or breadmaker on the unit where residents live.

This is the time to pet a cat and walk barefoot in the grass or dabble your feet in a pool. It is also the time to listen to music, maybe the same beloved piece over and over again. This is the time to look at big pictures of familiar, engaging, or simply beautiful things; or to watch children in the playground; or to hold hands and listen to a friendly voice saying something that sounds kind and nice. When a person can no longer understand the words being said, the sound of a familiar, comforting voice may be more precious than ever before.

It is also time to liven up the person's food, to add textures, flavor, aroma, and color. Unfortunately, most people's diets gradually degenerate into a saltless, textureless monotony. If no salt is to be added, then why not add oregano, savory, sweet basil, thyme, or sage? Pureeing food constitutes a serious deprivation and must be taken very seriously. Decorating a dish with garnishes and serving foods of different colors together is considered important in restaurants. It is no less important to the person for whom the meal may be the sensory highlight of the day.

Movement and rhythm are senses that require no interpretation to provide pleasure. Dancing, foot-stomping, hand-clapping, and drum-banging all produce wonderful sensations. Swings, hammocks, and rockers or gliders give the sensation of movement to people who can no longer move themselves. They also provide an alternative to people who move themselves so much that they wear out their caregivers.

Feeling and Expressing Emotions

Experiencing emotions and expressing emotion toward others are vital parts of human existence. Sometimes the dementing illness alters the manner in which the person experiences and exhibits his emotions. It can be either with a *flat affect,* no emotional expression at all, or *emotional lability,* the variable and occasionally explosive expression of emotions. Most people are somewhere between these extremes. Nonetheless, even the most impaired people need to express their emotions and respond to the emotions of others. This need is not limited to pleasant and positive emotions. It also includes sadness, anger, jealousy, frustration, and irritation. The full range is important.

This was brought home to me acutely during a small, nondirected group program I facilitated for five severely impaired residents of a nursing home. My habit was to empty a bag of various interesting articles on the table and invite these five residents to join me and see what I had brought. There was no discussion; I simply let the participants explore and handle the articles as they pleased and interact as they wished. This was only the third or fourth time we had met, so until then there had been very little interaction among the participants. This week the bag contained, among other things, a sheaf of wheat, a candle, a picture of a young man, a brownie pin, and a piece of white lace. One lady picked up the lace, looked at it for a while, and then put it to her face and started to cry. Her sobbing troubled me because I felt somehow responsible. Not knowing where this emotion had come from, I did not know what to do. The other members of the group did not know where her emotion had come from either, but they knew exactly what to do. They rallied around her, patted her back and comforted her. They experienced and shared a rare and very meaningful moment. We found out later, from her family, that this lady had been left at the altar as a young woman. She had not spoken of it for decades. None of the participants recalled the incident in the following weeks, but the group seemed, at least to me, to have greater cohesion.

Following a Logical Train of Thought

The last item on our list of retained abilities probably takes many readers by surprise. Many lists of disabilities associated with Alzheimer's disease include "the inability to think logically." The cognitively impaired person seems not to be thinking logically because his thought process leads him to conclusions that we do not perceive as logical. This happens because his logical reasoning is based on faulty information. Poor memory and attention span make it difficult for him to relate to recent events accurately and to handle several steps of the problem in sequence. However, the ability to see logical associations is very often intact. Given the correct information, one step at a time, the person can usually follow.

By the same token, the conclusions reached from reasoning that relies on memory of recent events and deals with many bits of information at once or in quick succession will seem, to him, patently illogical. That is what so often causes the cognitively impaired person to resist the good advice of his caregivers. The story of Mr. Y. in Chapter 2 is an example of exactly that situation. His information consisted of the following: He is an independent, competent adult. He lets his daughter do the laundry because he had never learned how to do it and at this stage in his life does not see the point of starting. However, he manages everything else to his satisfaction. The introduction of an in-home helper is, therefore, totally illogical. Hence his resistance.

Recognizing this capacity of the person to see the logical connection between ideas can help us accomplish more than one end. It lets us work with the person to achieve realistic solutions. A word of caution is needed, though. It would be a serious error to believe that the matter is settled once the person has agreed to a particular course of action or accepted a particular decision. This person also probably has a severe memory deficit and will not remember what he agreed to or the promises he made. The process will, most likely, have to be repeated many times before the resolution sticks. However, each time the process is repeated, it achieves another and equally important end. Our demonstration of respect and regard for the person reinforces the positive, collaborative relationship. Here is a story about how repetition finally paid off.

Mr. W. had been a longshoreman. He was big and burly, but a gentle and caring husband and father. He had initially been referred to our clinic because of impulsive and frequently abusive behavior toward his family. Cognitive testing revealed a moderate degree of dementia, and a physical examination revealed a severe gastric problem about which he had never complained. It needed surgical intervention and must have been quite painful. Mr. W. recovered from surgery very well, his behavior settled down, but his memory remained very poor. The dementia became more apparent now that he was no longer fighting and shouting. Despite that, things remained quite manageable. The stomach surgery somehow stayed in his mind as the commencement of his memory problems. He and his wife continued quite well until she became ill with cancer, which progressed very quickly. While Mr. W.'s wife was ill, they had in-home nursing and housekeeping. Mr. W. helped out and functioned very nicely. When she died, however, the services were removed and Mr. W. was on his own.

He did not cope well at all. Fortunately, the social worker who had taken his case from the first referral had established and maintained a sound relationship with both Mr. W. and his wife. Now that relationship proved invaluable. Mr. W. was threatened with eviction by the housing authority because he had burned his mattress. Efforts to move him into a care facility met with serious resistance. Everyone who came into the apartment—his son, the building superintendent, his sisters—all tried to convince him that he had to move. From his perspective they were all telling him something patently illogical. He had always been independent. Just because his wife was dead did not mean that he had to "move in with a lot of old people." Mr. W. was missing a vital bit of information in his reasoning—the fact that he had a severe memory problem.

The social worker drew up a plan in which all who were concerned about Mr. W. would enlist his capacity for logical thought. They would all visit more often to keep a closer eye on him but also to increase the frequency of the message. The line of reasoning that they would all use with him was as follows: "I am your friend [sister, buddy, son, etc.]. We usually see eye-to-eye. You trust me. I know you've always been a hard worker and are an intelligent man. After you had that stomach surgery [the point that Mr. W. could consistently identify] your memory was never the same. Remember how Alice had to take over the finances? When she was sick you took good care of her. But when she died, it was very hard on you. Look around. This place just doesn't look the same as it used to. I think you would be smart to move into a place where they would take care of these things for you. You deserve it."

Each person encountering Mr. W. would follow this line with him and would stop at the first sign of distress by simply saying "Okay" and letting the matter be. All sense of urgency about getting Mr. W. to move was dropped. Mr. W. was intelligent and could follow each step. Although he agreed that it would make sense to move, he had another solution. "I'll be okay," he would insist. "I will get over this. I have dealt with worse. All I need is to get back on my feet and I'll be fine." The social worker coached everyone to say something to the effect that they hoped, for his sake, that he would manage because it was hard to see him in this condition, that they would be available to him if he needed help, and just leave it at that.

The first break came not too long after the plan had been instituted. Mr. W. shifted his logic. He agreed with his son that it might be a good idea to just go and look at one of these places because he was really getting lonely. The son called the social worker. She arranged to have lunch with Mr. W. at one of the residential facilities that had a bed available. When she arrived to fetch Mr. W., he had forgotten the plan and his loneliness, and refused to go.

The social worker took a rain check on lunch. However, a step was added to the logical line of reasoning. Whenever Mr. W. mentioned his loneliness, the line that everyone included now was, "That's right, you had a chance to go with Sarah to have lunch and look at a nice place, but you turned it down." Mr. W. usually said something to the effect that that had not been very smart. The person would then let him know that he always had the option to make another appointment. Not long after, Mr. W. agreed to go again, but once more backed down at the last minute.

On the third try, Mr. W. made it to lunch. When he was introduced at the table, one of the ladies made a rhyme with his first name. "Walter, Walter will you take me to the altar?" Mr. W. agreed that any place where he could get a good meal and a marriage proposal on the same day could not be bad. He returned home that afternoon, packed his suitcase, and moved into the residential home.

This would seem, to some, to have been a lengthy and expensive intervention. But the alternative would have been no less expensive in both human and monetary costs. Mr. W. would have been removed forcibly from his apartment under a psychiatric commitment for endangering his life and those of others. He was a big man, given to defending his rights with his fists. He would have had to be sedated. If he had settled into the psychiatric ward routine and passed competency testing, he would have had to be released after the legal holding period for a psychiatric assessment had elapsed. If not, he would have had to be moved to a chronic ward to wait for admission into a long-term care facility. This whole process, the sedation and the loss of appropriate social context, would probably have unsettled him so much that he would not have been able to function in a residential home. He would have required skilled nursing care in a secured facility. As it happened, he spent three good years in residential care before being moved to a secure facility.

There are also times when the capacity for logic just gets in the way of a good time and is best put aside. We were getting ready to go out on a picnic, waiting for the last program participant to arrive. One of the gentlemen spotted the late arrival, a lady who always carried a tidy little handbag. There had been some talk about the weather. He said, "I hope you've brought us some sunny weather." She looked at her little bag a bit doubtfully and said, "This bag is too small. I couldn't bring much." Another gentleman who seemed not to have been listening at all, commented, "Well, if we take good care of it, it might grow." "How can you make sunny weather grow?" asked the voice of reason. To which a voice of even better reason answered, "Sprinkle sunshine all over the place. Put on a happy face!"

Other Important Personal Characteristics

It would be a great mistake to disregard the seventy to eighty years of life experience that have gone into building an individual personality and personal history. Chapter 3 elaborates on gathering history. This section looks at using that information to promote the best possible function and prevent challenging behavior; remember, the aim is not to change but to make the best use of what is there, which includes the person's

- identity, status, and role;
- values, ideals, prejudices, and personal ethic; and
- life experiences that form habits, memories, and fears.

Identity reflects who a person perceives herself as being. How often we see the cognitively impaired person looking at a picture of herself with no sense of recognition. This person may not see herself as the plump, cuddly, old lady in the picture. Perhaps she knows herself as a no-nonsense, efficient business manager. When pictures of residents are used to identify their rooms, it helps staff and visitors to use a current picture. It helps residents to use a picture of themselves that they recognize. This picture will also most accurately reflect that person's sense of identity.

Identity is also closely associated with one's professional and personal achievements. One lady on moving into a nursing facility was told to bring three pictures to hang on her wall. She chose a picture of her husband, one of her children, and her medical certificate. She said that she wanted to feel close to her family, but she also wanted to make sure that the people who came into her room knew how to treat her. This is the key. For unless we know who a person really is, we do not know how to treat her. When we fail to treat a person in a manner that is consistent with her identity, we can create problems. Once we know who this person really is, we have that necessary base on which we can establish a meaningful relationship. We also have a valuable tool that can affect the person's deportment. In one long-term care facility in the Czech Republic, the staff conducted a small experiment. They started consistently addressing the residents in one unit by their title, not only Mister, Mistress, and Doctor, but also Professor, Mr. Engineer, Mrs. Directress as was the custom among Czechs and other Europeans before World War II. They found a considerable degree of change in the general deportment of the staff and residents of that unit. Unpleasant behaviors and noise diminished. Pleasant social interactions increased. The equivalent, though perhaps not as dramatic in an Anglophone cultural context, would be the appropriate use of *Mr.* and *Mrs., Ms., Dr.,* and *Sir.*

Status reflects how one sees oneself in relation to others. Is this person accustomed to taking direction or giving it? Is this person accustomed to doing things or seeing to it that they get done? This will determine how we approach the person. It will also determine how we interpret program objectives with respect to each person. For example, we are committed to fostering autonomy and mastery. For one resident this might mean being able to tidy her own room. For another, it might mean watching someone else tidy and making sure that it is done to her satisfaction. To yet another it might mean having the room tidied regularly, to her standards, and with the least possible amount of attention from her. Although this objective relates to each of these three women, its realization must be individually determined with respect to the individual status of each.

The way a person will perceive his relationship with his caregiver will also be a function of status. This relationship should be based on trust and respect and should also accommodate the person's self-concept. Depending on the person's habitual status, the caregiver might seem to be a grandchild, an employee, a partner, a friend, an advisor, or a boss. It is not uncommon to hear caregivers introduced by these or similar terms. Whatever view of the relationship gives the person the most comfort is the one that is likely to be the most effective. There is nothing wrong with any of them as long as they reflect the person's preferred status.

Role reflects what the person believes he is meant to do with and for others. Is this person a leader or a follower? A helper? A counselor? A dependent? An organizer? Knowing a person's habitual role gives us another insight into how to treat her and what opportunities should be made available to her. The person who has always depended on others to take the lead and make decisions may not be comfortable when offered choices. A person who has been the one to make decisions will not take kindly to being told what to do. Yet both will function well if approached from their area of strength. It is not uncommon for programs serving persons with Alzheimer's disease to accommodate any number of CEOs, participants who engage in few of the activities, but pleasantly walk about congratulating staff and residents on their good work.

> The staff of one facility were very concerned about Mr. F., who was having much difficulty settling in. He was very distressed, asking anyone whom he saw why they were keeping him there. No activities suited him. He neglected his self-care even though he was capable. He had been by profession, and still was in life, a supervisor. The staff enlisted the help of the administrator, who came by each day before leaving the facility and asked Mr. F. how he felt things were going and what, if anything, could be done to improve things. Usually the reports were good and the main advice was to keep things just as they were. Mr. F. spent the rest of his days at the home, happily keeping an eye on things and making his reports. Occasionally he warned the staff that he would report something. They thanked him for making sure that standards were being maintained so well.

Knowledge of a person's values, ideals, prejudices, and personal ethic can help caregivers avoid problems. Many problems are caused when the residents' or participants' "dated" outlooks on issues as diverse as privacy, modesty, interior decorating, race and gender issues, or manners conflict with the more modern outlooks of the caregivers. Racial and religious prejudices are conditions with which many residents grew up and which, despite the current ethic, many have retained. They are not likely to change and so must be accommodated however possible. Individual perceptions must also be taken into consideration. If we find out that a gentleman is very concerned about "manliness," we will ask him whether he would prefer the help of a male or a female attendant in matters of intimate care. Perhaps this is a question that should be asked routinely. Even if we cannot do anything to change a situation, being able to acknowledge and accept the person's perspective is a valuable step toward coping with it. See Chapter 9 for more discussion of win-win communication.

Life experiences have formed the habits, memories, and fears that determine how a person interacts with her environment. We cannot change these influences. We must, however, know as much as possible about them. If we do, we can make the best use of them and avoid the problems that might arise from conflicts. There is a huge diversity of experience, even in a group in which the culture is relatively homogenous. It is ridiculous, therefore, to think that there is one schedule or standard protocol that will serve everyone well. It is little wonder that behavioral problems ensue when we try to force a fit. We might also be overlooking a treasure by not paying better attention to some old habits. In a tea group similar to the one described in Chapter 12, I tried to preserve an orderly and genteel atmosphere by encouraging the ladies to pass tea things nicely to one another. Once the group members became comfortable enough to let their old habits show, however, uniformly genteel behavior became less possible. One day a woman who had been a waitress at a truck stop took all the spoons from me and briskly tossed them around the table in front of each member, saying, "There you go, dearie. Here's one for you, sweetheart," and so on around the table. At first her manner took everyone by surprise. Once they all became accustomed to her, however, it became a kind of ritual that everyone in the group enjoyed. We thanked Alice for her lively contribution. Alice so loved to set and clear tables, and did it with such spirit, that it became her daily assignment in the dining room and a delight to everyone who saw her doing it.

In the face of a progressive illness that relentlessly erodes skills, memories, and knowledge, whatever remains becomes more and more valuable. There is really nothing that can be discarded as irrelevant.

8 | Responding to Problematic Behavior: A Process

The preceding two chapters examined ways of optimizing relationships and settings to prevent the most commonly recurrent problematic behaviors; this chapter presents a process of systematically looking at specific behaviors. The process involves four steps: (1) define the problem clearly and state specifically why it is a problem; (2) describe the circumstances that contributed to the problem and determine which of these can and should be changed; (3) develop a plan of intervention; and (4) evaluate and adjust the intervention. Before looking at the process, however, it is useful to look closely at the behavior that is considered problematic, why it is so considered, and what the aims of behavior management should be.

Some Perspectives on Problematic Behavior

Not All Seemingly Abnormal Behaviors Need Become Problems

Some problems are resolved simply by relabeling them as idiosyncrasies. The lady who insists on wearing three layers of clothing on hot summer days distresses those who think she is uncomfortable, but if it does not trouble her or put her physically in danger, it is not a problem. The gentleman who sits in the car for hours at a time might be finding comfort there. As long as he does not insist on driving, it is not a problem.

Other abnormal behaviors are manifestations of the person's disability and only become problems if we try to make the person behave as though the Alzheimer's disease did not exist. A question such as, "How do we get a person with a very short attention span to sit through a whole meal?" indicates a misplaced objective. The implied intent here is to change the person when it should be to change the circumstances. If we provide him with meals that can be eaten in stages, or "on the run," the problem ceases to exist. Another example is repetitive questioning. This becomes a problem behavior only when the caregiver, who does not understand the mechanism behind it, persists in efforts to make it go away.

Problems Exist in a Context

Some behaviors may become problems because of the context in which they occur. Nighttime wakefulness is one in particular. In a care facility, where fresh staff come on in the evening and can occupy and supervise a night owl, it is not a problem. A sole family caregiver, however, is very soon worn out by lack of sleep. Whereas it may be imperative to readjust a person's sleep habits in the home situation, there may be no real urgency to do so in a long-term care facility, unless, of course, the nighttime wakefulness is a sign of another underlying problem.

Not All Difficult Behavior Is Abnormal

We will never be able to prevent or eliminate all behaviors that make us uncomfortable, nor should we ever feel compelled to. Persons with cognitive impairment are individuals before all, and individuals have different ways of reacting to things. Their most effective means of coping may not always be the most comfortable for their caregivers. For example, roommates argue. Although there are times when the grievances are valid and must be rectified, there are other times when there is no real grievance. It is just their way of dealing with each other. Even though their behavior may be distressing to care providers, the two ladies who seem so antagonistic to one another would not want to live apart. Were they living in the community, they would probably be fighting over the back fence.

It Is Not Our Mandate to Change People

The aim of care is not to teach people to behave by their care providers' standards; it is to allow them to be themselves under the best possible circumstances. If a person's social competency, for example, is not evident, it is either because circumstances do not evoke it or because it is not recognized. In the first instance, our challenge as care providers is to create the circumstances in which the person is able to use his competencies. This has been the focus of the previous two chapters. In the second, the challenge is to see competent behavior in terms of the person's standards and not in terms of our own.

There will always be people who are difficult to live with. For some, rough manners and coarse language are simply their way of being. Others have been demanding, cantankerous and egocentric for many years.

This is how life has taught them to behave, and it has often served them well for seventy to ninety years. Morton Leiberman studied aged survivors of extreme adversity and found that, for the most part, they shared a singularly demanding, tenacious, egocentric, and cantankerous disposition. This was likely one of the factors that enabled them to come through those difficult situations. Most of the persons whom we encounter in long-term care are, above all, survivors.

In such cases, caregivers can only steel themselves and learn how to avoid altercations while protecting their own feelings. Distressed staff often say, "I don't have to take that kind of talk from her!" There is a simple answer: "You are absolutely right, you don't have to take it. She might hand it out, but you don't have to pick it up. So don't. Just leave it there." Any effort that a caregiver makes, either to defend himself or to correct the person, will only add fuel to the fire and breed antagonism between the two. Worst of all, it will undermine all other efforts to establish a relationship of trust. The best alternative is to acknowledge the person's upset and move politely to another topic. If that is not effective, it is best to simply leave; if leaving is not possible and nothing else has worked, politely let the person know that you are not going to react. A useful phrase is, "I am sorry that you feel that way."

Caregivers Need Support

The tolerance and insight that the above kind of response demands of a caregiver cannot be expected to come about on its own. Even if the caregiver comes to the caring situation with sensitivity and wisdom, he or she needs the support of education and counseling to maintain that perspective without burning out. The capacity to withstand harsh or insulting words, threats, and accusations, even if their source is understood, does not persist in a vacuum. It needs constant nurturing. Support services for caregivers, both family and paid care providers, are an essential component of any successful dementia care program.

Labeling a Behavior Can Hide the Real Problem

The term *aggressive behavior* is used to describe so many different behaviors that can each stem from so many different causes that it would be ridiculous to try to apply one intervention to them all. Yet, by labeling a person's action "aggressive behavior" we immediately imply that the person is engaging in an undesirable behavior that is a problem and must be stopped. The person who is doing whatever is labeled "aggressive behavior" can actually be

- defending himself,
- paying someone back,
- letting someone know that he has had enough,
- telling someone he is in pain, or
- protecting something precious.

In none of these cases would it be appropriate or effective to try to stop the behavior. The only solution is to identify and stop whatever he feels

- is attacking him,
- started it,
- is antagonizing him,
- is hurting him, or
- is threatening him.

"Wandering" and "sexually inappropriate" behavior are other such labels. Wandering can actually be

- going to work every day as you did for the past sixty years,
- escaping from an uncomfortable place,
- looking for something interesting,
- looking for something familiar, or
- feeling that you must be needed elsewhere because you are obviously not needed here.

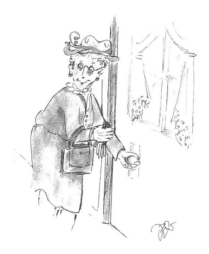

Going out, or is this wandering?

"Sexually inappropriate" behavior can be

- needing to touch and be touched,
- getting someone's attention,
- not remembering what to do or say when you are nervous and instead just blurting something out,
- mistaking a stranger for the person with whom you are normally intimate,
- wanting to be with someone special, and
- wanting to be special to someone.

This is not to suggest that none of these behaviors constitutes a problem. It means that classifying them under a stock label conceals the actual nature of what is going on.

Not All Settings Can Respond Effectively to All Difficult Behaviors

There are some persons whose combination of severe cognitive and psychiatric disorders requires specialized settings and treatment. These are people whose needs exceed the resources of most in-home caregivers, day care centers, or conventional long-term care facilities. All community counselors and program operators have a responsibility to identify these persons' needs, and to direct them to the facilities that can serve them best.

There Are No Quick Solutions

There can be no universal troubleshooting list or recipe file of solutions to problematic behaviors, because one behavior pattern can have any number of precipitators and each will demand a different intervention. The danger of lists or recipe files is that they promote a cookie-cutter approach instead of real problem solving. Although a prescribed intervention may sometimes resolve a problem, in the long run it will create even more problems and frustrations. Even if it works, the caregiver may not really understand why, and so will not know whether it can be applied to other situations or how to make adjustments if the intervention ceases to be effective. If the approach does not work, the caregiver is liable to feel frustrated and conclude that the problem is unsolvable. This is discouraging and contributes to the caregiver's feelings of helplessness and burnout.

There is, however, a process that puts the caregiver into a partnership with the cognitively impaired person, and helps them determine the best solution for both. The process involves active problem definition, information gathering, a review of resources, and the evolution of a plan. This approach has the added benefit of giving the caregiver a way of seeing the problem as a puzzle to be solved instead of a trial to be endured. It places tools in the caregiver's hands that will eventually be applicable to many other situations.

This method is also useful in that it keeps the problem-solving process going until a rational resolution is achieved. It also promotes an active investigation that may uncover problems that would not have been suspected otherwise. One lady was severely misbehaving at the table. In the course of the problem-solving process, a number of medical issues, including dental problems and a hiatus hernia, were discovered that would not have been identified if the focus had remained exclusively on her shouting and throwing food.

The Process

An exercise illustrating this process is found in Exhibit 4.

Gathering Information to Put Things in Perspective

Before we can begin to formulate a solution to any behavior, we have to know the situation, get the facts, and clearly define the problem. An attempt to alter anyone's behavior without finding out exactly what is going on can be not only ineffective but also injurious. It denies the person's individuality and assumes incompetence.

Without such information, caregivers who have been having an especially difficult time with a cognitively impaired person may be inclined to attribute the behavior to willfulness and malicious intent. They may conclude on the basis of "gut feelings," for example, that refusal to eat is attention seeking or that resistance to care is due to hostility.

We should be able to answer the following questions before we decide to do anything. Let us use them as a guide to examine the situation of Mr. L. He is a resident of a nursing home, is being physically and verbally abusive to staff, and is resisting care. It takes two people to hold him down while another changes his incontinence pad. He has been in the home for five years because of dementia. For the last two years, after having had a stroke, he has used a wheelchair. He has limited use of his left side.

These are the questions to which we must respond.

EXHIBIT 4. A PROBLEM-SOLVING EXERCISE

When a person behaves in a manner that causes concern to care providers, he is usually doing the best he can under difficult circumstances. He usually is unable to explain the reason for his behavior or offer alternatives. The onus of resolving the situation, therefore, lies with us. Here is a format that can lead us through the problem-solving process.

Gather Information

(If some facts are not available, make them up for this exercise, but note the need to find them out.)

- Describe the behavior.
- What makes this behavior a concern?
- Is it significantly different from the person's previous behavior? How?
- Whom does the behavior affect adversely?
- When does the behavior occur? Where? How often?
- Who else is involved in the incidents?
- What are the circumstances leading up to the behavior?
- Do the circumstances in any way conflict with the person's values, needs, habits, or convictions? How?
- What aspects of the person's mental impairment or medical condition contribute to the behavior?
- What aspects of the nonhuman environment contribute?
- What aspects of the human environment contribute?
- How does the person feel about the incidents?

Define the Problem

- Has our view of the original problem changed? How?
- What is the problem?
- What would we like to see as an alternative?
- What would the person like to see as an alternative?

Design the Plan

- How can the person change to achieve this alternative?
- Considering the resources available, is this realistic?
- How can the person's nonhuman environment be changed to achieve this alternative?
- Considering the resources available, is this realistic?
- How can the person's human environment be changed to achieve this alternative?
- Considering the resources available, is this realistic?

State the Plan

- What will be done?
- Who will be involved?
- When?
- How?
- For how long?

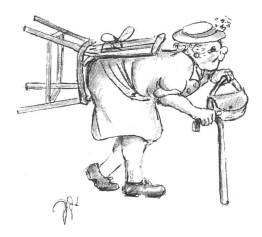

"Port-a-chair"

How would you describe the behavior in objective terms, making no assumption about motive or intent? This is our first challenge. Mr. L. demonstrates so many behaviors that are a concern and staff have become so frustrated by trying to care for him that they produce a litany of problem behaviors whenever his name is mentioned. We must concentrate on one behavior at a time, even though several may be linked and they all need attention. For the purpose of this exercise, we will focus on his resisting personal care. The behavior is stated as "resisting the approach of caregivers while they try to perform personal care," not "being hostile to staff during care."

What makes this behavior a concern? Is it problematic because of its effect on the person himself, on the people around him, on his environment, or on the observer? The answer to this question determines the extent to which an actual behavioral change is needed. There are many reasons why Mr. L.'s behavior is a concern. Staff are afraid of him and are distressed at having to do things to him while he screams and tries to hit them. The sound of his struggle distresses other residents. Most of all, staff realize how disturbed he must be to be fighting so hard for so long.

When, where, with whom, how often, and how long does this behavior happen? It is often useful to chart observations for some time to see if a pattern emerges. A sample format for documenting such observations can be found in Exhibit 5. In this case, the behavior happens each time any personal care is required because there is already a pattern in place.

EXHIBIT 5. BEHAVIOR DOCUMENTATION FORM

Person's Name ___Mrs. L.___ Room ___440B___ Observation period ___03/06___ to ___8/06___

Date	Time	Place	Other Person(s) Involved	Circumstances Leading to the Incident	Description of the Incident	Intervention Tried, If Any	Outcome of Intervention	Initial of Observer
03/06	08:30	Dining room	Mrs. K.	Mrs. K. wanted to sit in Mrs. L.'s chair.	Mrs. K. said it was hers. Mrs. L. poked her with her cane.	I brought Mrs. L. to her room and told her not to do that.	Mrs. L. shouted in her room for 10 minutes, then fell asleep.	JP
04/06	08:10	Hallway 4B	Mr. G.	Mrs. L. was in Mr. G.'s room. He shouted at her to get out.	Mrs. L. said it was her room and raised her cane at him.	I brought Mrs. L. to her room and told her not to do that.	She shouted in her room for 10 minutes, then fell asleep.	KL
06/06	07:55	Dining room	Mrs. J.	Mrs. L. said Mrs. J. had her sweater. Mrs. J. said no, it's mine.	Mrs. L. demanded to have it and jabbed at Mrs. J. with her cane.	I explained to Mrs. L. that it was not her sweater and that she should not hit.	She said she was tired and everyone was taking her things. She wanted to go to her bedroom.	JP
08/06	08:05	Hallway 4B	Mr. G.	Mrs. L. was in Mr. G.'s room. He shouted at her to get out.	Mrs. L. said it was her room and threatened to hit him with her cane.	I took Mrs. L. to her room.	She lay down and cried, then fell asleep.	JP

Three staff members approach Mr. L. when they intend to change his pad. As soon as he sees this, he stiffens and starts to shout. The staff feel they have no choice but to force him into compliance, since he is already struggling and resisting even before they try to lift him from his chair onto the bed.

What are the consequences of the behavior to the person, to those around him, to his caregiver, and to his environment? Everyone fears him. He is very angry and obviously suffering. His hygiene is also suffering. The situation is getting progressively worse.

How does the person react to these consequences? He is becoming more and more resistant. He does not seem to understand what is going on. He just fights blindly. His only utterances are abusive exclamations. He is becoming more withdrawn.

Is the behavior directly related to aspects of the person's cognitive impairment? Often the problem arises from unrealistic expectations being placed on a cognitively impaired person who is unable to perform. When that is the case, expectations or requirements must change. This is where gaps in staff knowledge of Mr. L. appear. They do not know his cognitive state, how much he understands, or how much he would be able to cooperate if he were not fighting. They are caught in a reactive cycle. Because they are not aware of his limitations, they expect cooperative behavior from him and attribute his resistance to hostility. New staff seem to get along with him better at first, possibly because they do not know him very well and tend to approach him more slowly and quietly. This might be what he needs. We do know that Mr. L. has moderate to severe dementia, as well as perceptual problems, especially with things on his left side, related to his stroke. Some staff notice that he is more likely to be startled when approached from the left side. None of this is documented and none of this information figures in his management plan.

Is the behavior directly related to a superimposed medical condition? A cognitively impaired person may be less able to cope or explain the effect of some other condition that is causing pain, discomfort, or functional loss. Mr. L. has a subluxation (partial dislocation) of his left hip and has arthritis, both of which might be causing pain, especially when he is lifted. Neither of these issues figures in his care plan. His balance is very poor, and he may be afraid of falling. His left side is weak, and he may feel insecure, especially when held by two people he does not trust.

What aspects of the human environment contribute? The staff's approach, we see now, is a trigger. Whether we think that things could be done any other way is immaterial. The fact remains that the approach of three people is threatening.

What aspects of the nonhuman environment contribute? Staff report that they feel rushed. Because they anticipate that Mr. L.'s change will take a lot of time, they feel pressured even before engaging him. The scheduled and task-oriented way of working that is part of the facility's system contributes to the problem. Staff need to feel that they can give Mr. L. more time. They also notice that his bedroom is oriented so that people coming in are approaching him on his left and vulnerable side. The grab bar in his room is on the left, and therefore not very useful to him; because of this positioning he is unable to assist in his own transfer.

Does this behavior differ from the person's lifelong pattern in responding to similar circumstances? If so, how? The staff know little of Mr. L.'s past. They do know that he was a businessman. It is therefore likely that this behavior differs from his habitual way of acting. The circumstances, however, also differ from anything to which he may have been accustomed. If he is reacting to being held down by two people who are hurting him while a third removes his underwear, perhaps he is not being altogether unreasonable.

How does the person feel about the behavior, the circumstances leading to it, and the consequences of it? Too often the central figure in this whole affair is left out. An interview with Mr. L. reveals that his vocabulary is very limited. He is very sad and feels isolated. He has only one friend in the world, who seldom visits. He is angry with the staff, considers them rude, and feels that they are hostile to him. When a new staff member comes on he hopes for a friend and, in his words, "Then they all turn out to be the same."

Do the circumstances in any way conflict with the person's values, needs, habits, or convictions? How? The available information about Mr. L. suggests that the circumstances as described above are an affront to him.

A very important outcome of this process is that, by this point, caregivers find out they really do not have enough information. This is a very important realization because it underscores how little information we usually have before embarking on a plan. It is little wonder, then, that our plans fail to hit the mark so often. Another important outcome of this information-gathering exercise is that it forces the caregiver to examine the situation closely from the cognitively impaired person's perspective. This process in itself has the effect of fortifying the relationship or, in this case, helping staff to realize that there is no positive relationship, which in itself is likely to be contributing to the problem.

In some cases, this exercise helps the caregiver understand the source of the behavior and eventually to tolerate it, thus eliminating the need to change it. In this case, although the staff might understand Mr. L.'s situation better, they cannot merely tolerate his behavior. The staff sees now how their lack of knowledge and unilateral approach are contributing to the problem. This insight helps to redefine the problem. Mr. L. does not trust them. They do not know him, nor do they credit him with any ability to cooperate. There is one small opening that they could exploit, his stated hope each time that a new staff member might be a friend.

Stating the Objective

Define the problem. Has our view of the original problem changed? How? What is the problem? Now we see the problem differently. There is a lack of knowledge, mutual trust, and respect. The combative behavior is not occurring in isolation and is not even really the principal problem.

What would we like to see as an alternative? Although we would ultimately like to see Mr. L. cooperate with personal care, we need to get to know him and establish trust.

What would the person like to see as an alternative? Mr. L. has already told us what he would like—a friend.

Designing the Plan

How can the person change to achieve this alternative? Considering the resources available, what is realistic? Mr. L. cannot change on his own. He is already doing the best he can.

How can the person's nonhuman environment be changed to achieve this alternative? Considering the resources available, what is realistic? His room can be rearranged to accommodate his unilateral disregard and weakness of the left side. We can also consider pain medication, a transfer process that will minimize discomfort, and proper seating to alleviate pain.

How can the person's human environment be changed to achieve this alternative? Considering the resources available, what is realistic? The staff are motivated to help Mr. L., but there is also a lot of animosity and resentment permeating their relationship. They need counseling to deal with that and adopt a positive outlook on him. Perhaps learning some of his background and previous achievements may help to build their esteem for him. Their interactions with him outside the personal care situation must be used to build a positive relationship. They need a clear understanding of his cognitive ability and physical limitations. Occupational therapy assessment and interpretation would be helpful here. All this must be done with the resources available, but the situation, as it stands, is far too costly in terms of staff time and morale and Mr. L.'s well-being.

Stating the Plan

Now and only now are we ready to suggest a course of action. *What shall be done?* A plan may take any number of forms:

- It may be as simple as the caregiver's learning to accommodate to a behavior.
- It may require a change of routine, priorities, or setting, such as changing the attendant who provides personal care or changing the time of a person's bath.
- It may require a change in the caregiver's approach to a situation. In the case of Mr. L., we observed that a slow approach by one person at a time was better accepted.
- It may require a proactive approach in terms of instituting a program or situation that will address the patient's needs and avert or preclude the occurrence of the behavior in question. Examples include caregivers making a special effort to knock on the door and wait for an answer before entering a person's room, or asking a person to hand them the tray before taking it. In Mr. L.'s case, establishing a relationship in other contexts and learning about him will be important.
- It may require medication or medical treatment. In Mr. L.'s case, pain medication is a possibility. Medical intervention may also be necessary. A psychiatrist may need to prescribe a mild sedative to be administered before the pad change. This is what it may take to enable him to tolerate even the calm, slow approach at first. Gradually, as staff are able to gain his trust they will be able to do the change without medication. This is often the case when a severe behavior has been going on for a long time. It would be a grave mistake, however, to think that the medication itself is a solution. It is only an aid to enable the social intervention.
- It may require a series of progressive steps toward a goal. In this case, each step becomes a short-term goal. In the case of a client who acutely feared being bathed, the home visiting nurse had to slowly establish her trust and progressively ease her toward the bathtub. They started by talking about her aching feet, after which she agreed to do a foot soak in the kitchen; then they moved to the bathroom and started wetting more and more of her legs until she had to raise and eventually remove her skirt. Then they soaked

her feet in the bathtub and gradually moved to sponging and eventually tub bathing. Each time the goal was to move one step closer to the bath while maintaining the client's comfort and, hence, trust in the situation. In Mr. L.'s case, the change of an incontinence pad cannot be accomplished through a slow desensitization process, but the building of the relationship will need to proceed in small steps.

Who should be involved? Everyone is somehow implicated, and the role of each one must be clearly stated. In the case of Mr. L., all staff have a role to play in building his trust and learning about him. Those staff whom he mistrusts the least should be the ones who do his personal care.

When? There are some interventions for which the timing is important and must be clearly stated. In the case of Mr. L., pad changes can be scheduled for those times when he is least irritable or apprehensive, perhaps after meals.

For how long? Caregivers must be patient and committed to giving any intervention a good trial. Most problematic behaviors have been developing over many years, and it is not likely that they will be resolved in a matter of days or even weeks. In any consultation that our clinic did, we requested that the staff be committed to a six-week period, with an initial review after a three-week trial.

Implementing a Plan

Whatever the plan, it must be applied consistently and with commitment and persistence. Few things work the first time, especially with a cognitively impaired person whose memory for recent events is impaired, but who clings tenaciously to old habits. There are times when the institution of a plan actually seems to make the behavior worse. This is usually the case when the behavior is the consequence of broken trust and fear. The person does not know what is going on. He remains prepared, however, to defend himself. Only when the trusting relationship is reestablished can he relax his guard, and then we see improvement. It can take a long time.

Wherever possible, the solution must also involve the patient. We tend to underestimate the ability of a cognitively impaired person to relate to what we consider complex issues, and therefore leave them out of the planning and resolution of a problem. We mustn't forget that a cognitively impaired person remains sensitive to emotional matters, and needs reassurance, comfort, and an opportunity to feel that others understand and include him in decisions. In Mr. L.'s case, simply letting him know that staff were distressed with his reaction out of concern for him would make a difference in his perception of them. Even if he did not remember the information from one time to another, he would eventually come to feel the sentiment they were expressing.

It often helps to get professional assistance. A family caregiver is likely to be too close and emotionally involved to evaluate the situation impartially, and will need help and moral support to implement and follow through with a plan. Professional caregivers may have been involved in a long process of trial and error solutions, and may have become overwhelmed with a challenging problem. Often they need a guide to help them step back from the situation.

Evaluating Outcome, an Ongoing Process

Once the plan is devised, a process of evaluation must be put into place. It is useful to continue the behavior documentation form that was started at the beginning. This helps caregivers monitor their responses to the behavior, their consistency in implementing the intervention, and the person's response to the intervention.

If the intervention has the desired effect, it must be continued. Behavioral interventions are palliative in nature, not curative. They make the situation manageable. They do not make the underlying factors go away. If the intervention works very well, caregivers are apt to forget about it and revert to the old methods that may have spawned the problem in the first place. An analogy can be drawn with a chronic back problem. The physiotherapist will prescribe exercises and a special pillow. These interventions work so well and the patient feels so good that he stops doing the exercises and even puts away the special pillow. In no time at all the back problem returns. It is the same with behavioral interventions. They must become a long-term commitment. If the interventions with Mr. L. are effective, caregivers must remain vigilant that they do not slip back into the old ways of doing things. As new staff come on, they must also be informed of his background, his preferences, and the programs that work best for him.

If the intervention does not have the desired effect, or if it stops working, the process naturally starts again, building on and verifying the information that was collected the first time. This approach is a continuous process, not an ad hoc procedure that is called on to deal with a crisis. It is a standing method of clarifying, asking, accommodating, and being critically aware of what we are doing.

This process cannot be implemented in a vacuum; it must be supported by staff training and support programs. For it to be effective, staff must work as a team; this requires team building and maintenance on an ongoing basis.

Individual Responses to Problematic Behaviors

The process described in this chapter requires team commitment and effort. The team is, however, made up of individuals. Everyone has a responsibility to ensure that problematic behaviors are dealt with sensitively and effectively, and that they do not escalate into major crises. The following are guidelines for individual caregivers when they encounter a person engaging in difficult or problematic behavior.

To maintain a positive relationship that does not threaten the person's sense of control:

- Keep the person's attention by maintaining eye contact and a friendly, calm attitude.
- Don't ask questions or demand explanations about the behavior.
- Avoid criticizing or admonishing.
- Avoid a power struggle.
- Help the person save face.
- Identify and acknowledge emotions that the person is expressing.
- Identify a need which the person is expressing.
- Offer a reasonable alternative to the person, or, if that is not possible or acceptable, offer sympathy and divert or redirect the person to a more positive activity.

To prevent or minimize future occurrences of the problem:

- Identify what triggered the behavior.
- Identify your feelings about the behavior, and analyze how you dealt with them.
- Share this information with your team and identify permanent changes to the environment that could reduce the recurrence of similar incidents.

9 | Communication: The Heart of Relationships

"We have reached an agreement." "He doesn't understand me." "We've had a breakdown in communication." Even though these statements comment on communication, they all have to do with a relationship. At the core of every relationship, be it business, romantic, parental, marital, or caregiving, lies the ability of both parties to communicate. Alzheimer's disease profoundly affects communication at all levels and, with it, the relationship between the affected person and the caregivers. As the affected person's ability to communicate slips away, family caregivers often feel as though the relationship itself is slipping away. They experience the loss of the person even though he is still with them. If the relationship has been difficult to begin with, loss of communication can aggravate what is already a strained situation and broaden the rift. Problems with communication can hamper the formation of a new working relationship between professional caregivers and their cognitively impaired clients, keeping the person who is newly admitted to a residence or day program isolated and lonely.

Because the quality of life of both the affected person and those caring for him depends so much on the nature of their relationship, it is crucial that they maintain the best possible communication throughout the course of the person's illness. To achieve this, caregivers must understand the nature of the communication barriers that dementing illness can raise. This chapter collects ideas and information from other sections of the book and relates them directly to the issue of communication.

Communication consists of more than just the ability to exchange words; it is the ability to connect with someone. That requires comfort, security, and trust among the individuals involved. While Alzheimer's disease imposes specific language deficits and makes the exchange of words difficult, it also affects the person's capacity to cope with social and emotional situations. This chapter examines the emotional and social vulnerabilities that affect the cognitively impaired person's capacity to communicate, and offers strategies for preventing or defusing uncomfortable situations that could undermine a relationship. It also describes ways of coping with the specific language deficits most often associated with Alzheimer's disease.

When we feel a familiar relationship slipping away or when we have trouble establishing a new one, there is reassurance in knowing that there are things we can do to lessen the sense of separation. Many of the approaches offered here are simple, common sense. They are discussed because many are so natural to us that we may underestimate their value. Others may actually be contrary to our normal instincts and, therefore, may require some conscious practice, experimentation, and, in some cases, a good deal of courage.

As we know, few things work the first time we try them, and almost nothing works every time. But we have no way of knowing whether or not an approach will work until we try it. The objective is, first, to acquire a good understanding of what we are dealing with and, second, to furnish ourselves with a variety of strategies with which to approach the situation. This will go a long way to helping us gain control of the situation and perceive it as something we can influence. This is very important, because hopelessness and a feeling of impotence are the most debilitating barriers that a caregiver can face.

Principles of Effective Communication

We are more likely to establish and maintain effective communication with a cognitively impaired person if we keep in mind the following four principles:

- Cognitively impaired persons have special communication needs resulting from their emotional dependency and their inability to make concessions and accommodations.
- The responsibility for understanding and being understood lies with the caregiver.
- Our most important task is to establish and nurture a partnership of mutual trust and respect.
- The person we are working with has a real and persistent communication disability. Although we cannot make the disability go away, we can employ effective strategies to help overcome specific problems.

These principles are key to all the aspects of dementia care discussed in this book, so we'll look at each in more detail.

Special Communication Needs of Persons with Alzheimer's Disease

The special communication needs of persons with Alzheimer's disease come from the double blow that the disease inflicts. Not only does it make it very difficult for the affected person to function, but also it removes the insight and understanding that would enable him to cope with his disability. This leaves him unable to compensate and come to terms with the situation as he might with a physical disability. It creates a vulnerability that is at the heart of many of the difficult and challenging behaviors we see in persons with Alzheimer's disease.

Alzheimer's Disease and Emotional Dependency

The person who has little or no memory, who cannot analyze and understand complex information, is not only physically dependent on others, but also emotionally dependent. This kind of dependency may not always be obvious, but it has tremendous significance. It means that the person is reliant on his immediate environment and on the people around him for information, assurance, and guidance. Whatever message that environment provides is likely to be taken at face value, and will determine how he feels, and what he thinks of himself and the situations he finds himself in. If the message suggests that he is loved, respected, and safe, he is likely to feel that way. If the message is perceived as disquieting or provoking, the person is likely to feel uncomfortable or irritated. Every encounter is a fresh experience for the memory-impaired person. Therefore, with every encounter the caregiver influences, positively or negatively, how the cognitively impaired person feels.

Even an apparently trivial interchange can have a great impact. Take, for example, the situation of removing dirty cups and saucers from someone's place. It can be done without exchanging a word, perhaps even without making eye contact. It is done this way countless times every day in retirement homes, hospitals, and nursing homes. It does no obvious harm to anyone, yet there is a message here. The staff member's behavior implies, "I am busy. I have other things on my mind. My job is to keep this place tidy, and right now I'd rather you didn't obstruct me." A person with good memory, insight, and judgment can take that message for what it is worth and try not to take it personally. He might even wonder what is wrong and express concern for the staff person who is usually attentive and considerate.

This is because, under normal conditions, we take into consideration whatever we know about the person with whom we are speaking and their circumstances when we interpret what they are saying or not saying. We usually make this interpretation with good will toward the other person and confidence in our own value and standing. A person with Alzheimer's disease cannot remember or use such contextual information and, therefore, is vulnerable to the full impact of the most obvious and concrete message embedded within each encounter. The message that an emotionally dependent person might take from the above encounter is "You don't count. You are not important. You have no control here. You are useless."

Now let's imagine the encounter with the following dialogue:

> "Mrs. Jones, are you finished with your cup?"
> "Em hm."
> "Can you hand it to me, please?"
> "Here."
> "Thanks!"

In this tiny interchange, the message that the person is most likely to receive is "You can influence this situation. We acknowledge you. You are useful." Imagine the power of this message as it is repeated each time a caregiver needs to reach for something near the person, pass something by him or have him move over to let someone pass by or mop the floor. If we remain mindful of this emotional dependency during every encounter with a cognitively impaired person, we will be able to avoid many unpleasant situations and move a long way toward building a positive and respectful relationship.

There is, of course, always the chance that this approach will be met with a bitter, resentful response from an irritable, unhappy, or depressed person. He might tell the caregiver to "take it and get lost" or he might refuse to answer. Whatever the response, the caregiver knows that he has done his best. With consistency, the situation can only improve.

An Impaired Ability to Accommodate

A person with Alzheimer's disease is far less able to cope with or make allowances for the communication errors and oversights of others. In most of our relationships, we accommodate the poor communication skills of others and they, in turn, make allowances for our communication blunders. If you were to listen critically to a tape of a normal conversation, you would probably find that much of the information exchanged is quite inaccurate and incomplete. Our communication usually works despite these failings because we can rely on each other to fill in the gaps and adjust the inaccuracies with our insight and our ability to extrapolate. This flexibility is what makes our relationships work.

A person with Alzheimer's disease finds it difficult to grasp abstract ideas. He cannot "read between the lines," and so cannot make this leap into understanding. When bits of information are missing or the message is ambiguous a cognitively impaired person is easily confused. To try to make sense of things, he may impose his own interpretation onto the situation, most likely an interpretation that is dictated entirely by his internal state and that may have little or nothing to do with the actual circumstances. For example:

> Mrs. X.'s son and daughter-in-law have come to visit with the three grandchildren. They have decided to have a game of cards. Someone has asked Grandma where the cards are, but she is not sure. In fact, she hardly answered. So instead of bothering her any more, the youngsters set about looking through the drawers in the living room cabinets where they know she used to keep the cards.
>
> Mrs. X. really does not know what is going on. She is already nervous about having five people in the house at once. And she was always afraid for her porcelain figurines whenever the children came into the parlor. Now they are rummaging in the drawers. She has already lost so many lovely things. This makes her very uncomfortable, but she is too polite to say anything right now. As John and the grandchildren leave, Mrs. X. tells him that they are not welcome again because she knows that they have stolen things.

A series of unfortunate coincidences has conspired to create this terrible feeling in Mrs. X. Her family is devastated. If they can trace things back to the contributing factors, they can save themselves the pain of believing that their grandmother hates them or is hopelessly paranoid. Mrs. X. was overwhelmed by the number of people in her house. She did not grasp the reason for the search of her cabinets and therefore felt that her property was being violated. If the family can understand how vulnerable Mrs. X. is, next time they will not touch her things without her permission and might even invite her to participate in the search.

Because the person's interpretation of a situation may differ so markedly from ours, it may seem that his reactions are irrational and irrelevant. Such a conclusion is dangerous because it threatens our respect for the person and, hence, our relationship with him. Remember, all reactions are relevant, but some may be relevant to a set of circumstances that we do not understand or are not aware of.

Assuming Responsibility for Understanding and Being Understood

There is meaning behind everything that a cognitively impaired person says. A person with dementia is no more likely to spout nonsense now than he ever was. What may be unintelligible to us is not nonsense to the person who is saying it. He is doing his best to tell us something that has meaning and it is up to us to figure out what that meaning is.

We usually think of communication as a two-way street and a shared responsibility. In dealing with a person who has Alzheimer's disease, the responsibility for understanding and being understood lies squarely with the caregiver. It may seem to be a heavy burden, but it is one that is lightened by the knowledge that in assuming responsibility, we also gain control. We can take the lead, ask clarifying, yes-or-no questions, direct or redirect the conversation, or use visual prompts. When things are not going well, we can back off, express regret that we do not understand, and offer to try again later. If the person had the ability to make himself more clearly understood, he would have done so. We cannot expect any more effort from him than he is already giving. By taking control of the situation with skill and understanding, we can do much to avoid frustration and keep the relationship between ourselves and our clients or loved ones comfortable and mutually respectful.

We also take control by paying attention to how we initiate conversations and phrase questions. The most common traps into which caregivers fall are asking open-ended questions or expecting the person to make decisions which he is not capable of making. Once the question is asked, the caregiver has relinquished control and can only deal with the often negative consequences. Here are a few examples.

Early one morning, Mr. Y., still in his pajamas, is feeling restless and has a vague notion that he'd like to go out. He goes to the door, and his caregiver calls out, "Mr. Y., where are you going?" Now Mr. Y. is compelled to answer even if he had no clear intention of going anywhere specific—after all, a direct question demands a direct answer. He will likely respond with the first thing that comes to his mind. His answer will probably be drawn from old habits and routines, and will be so much in keeping with his nature that the caregiver will not question his intent. "I'm going to the bank. Won't be long," he calls back, and then he heads out the door. Now his caregiver becomes alarmed. Her tone of voice betrays her as she says, "No, Mr. Y., you can't go out now. We'll go out later, as soon as you get your clothes on." Mr. Y. is, however, already in the "going-to-the-bank" state of mind and is difficult to dissuade. In addition, if he has any inkling that he is trying to go to the bank in his pajamas, he will be terribly embarrassed and must now try to save face. Even if the situation is eventually resolved, an uncomfortable episode was initiated, albeit innocently, by the caregiver's open-ended question. With this question she inadvertently put Mr. Y. on the spot. She relinquished control of the situation to him, but he couldn't cope and just responded as best he could.

There would have been no lack of respect in the caregiver's maintaining control and offering Mr. Y. one or several viable alternatives such as "Do you want to see what it's like outside?" or "Let's see if the paper has come yet." She could also have distracted and redirected him with "Mr. Y., could you come here for a moment? I'd like you to help me with something." Any of these approaches might have avoided a conflictual situation and preserved Mr. Y.'s dignity, as well as the relationship with his caregiver.

On the other hand, Mr. Y. may already have been stewing over something else for a long time, and could have been bound and determined to leave. In that case, he might insist on going out in his pajamas, and the caregiver would have to either let him walk off or redirect him into the house with some plausible suggestion. In any event, there was nothing to be gained from that first open-ended question; it can only make the situation worse.

Mrs. K. was a socially active lady with a long-standing habit of lunching at the club, shopping, and visiting friends. She has become quite frail and can no longer sustain that pace. However, each time her caregiver asks her what she would like to do that day, her automatic answer is lunch at the club, shopping, or visiting a friend. After a day of being out, she is exhausted and evenings are very difficult. She might very well have enjoyed a ham sandwich at home, a game of cards, or a stroll in the garden. But because these activities are not part of her habitual repertoire, she is unable to suggest them when asked what she would like to do.

One day her caregiver, instead of asking Mrs. K. what she wants to do, suggests lunch on the patio or a game of cards. Mrs. K. readily agrees and has a good time. If Mrs. K. would rather have gone out to lunch, she still had the option to say so. If she did not want to play cards, she could let her caregiver know. In any case, however, Mrs. K.'s caregiver avoided putting her on the spot with a direct, open-ended question and discovered new options for her.

This is not to say that all stressful occurrences can be avoided or easily defused. It just means that if we consciously keep control of the situation, working with and not against the person's abilities and deficits, we can do a lot to avoid many recurrent stressors and safeguard that all-important relationship between ourselves and the dependent person.

Aim to Establish or Maintain a Partnership

From the very start, things will be easier if the cognitively impaired person knows that the two of you are in this together, that he can trust you, that you respect him, and that you will always be there for him. Although such an alliance may seem nearly impossible to establish in some cases, it is actually easier than it seems. The "we'll-lick-this-problem-together" approach is an effective tack to take in any potentially adversarial encounter. In fact, it also works very well with spouses, children, and colleagues. It is especially important in dealing with a person whose insight and judgment are impaired, because this person, confronted with someone he perceives as an adversary, naturally seeks to defend himself. On the other hand, he will, just as naturally, find comfort in an ally. The former situation creates a rift, while the latter binds a relationship.

Every potentially adversarial situation can be outlined as a triangle, with three elements: the client, the problem, and the caregiver. It need not be a very complicated or profound situation. For example, Mrs. X., who must be supervised with smoking materials, wants to have a cigarette. Joe, her caregiver, cannot leave what he is doing to accompany her and tells her so. The triangle is formed by Mrs. X., the fact that she cannot have a cigarette when she wants it (the problem), and Joe. In this case, the adversarial lines are drawn, in Mrs. X.'s mind, between Joe and herself by Joe's inadvertently allying himself with the problem when he refused to let her have a cigarette immediately. Now she has not only her nicotine craving to contend with, but also the fact that her caregiver won't help. She's annoyed, but can do nothing. Mrs. X. remembers Joe's explanation for two minutes and then asks for the cigarette again. She is told once again that she will not get what she wants. The adversarial lines intensify. This goes on until Joe either finds the time or gives in, or Mrs. X. forgets about the cigarette. Each time something like this happens, a small, perhaps insignificant, rift is created between Mrs. X. and her caregiver. If the relationship is otherwise sound, it may have

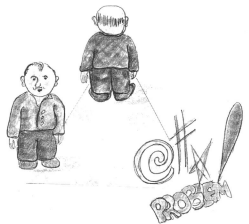

Every potentially adversarial situation has three elements: you, me, and the problem.

When one of us aligns himself with the problem and against the other, we create odds of two to one. This may start an argument and can threaten the relationship.

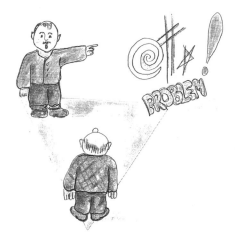

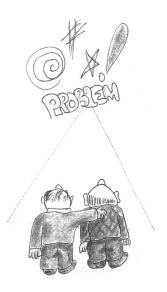

Win-win communication aligns us with the other person to create a team who will face the problem together. This strengthens the relationship.

no lasting consequences. But, if this sort of adversarial situation is repeated often enough, the cumulative effect may eventually taint their
relationship.

How could the situation be handled differently? Joe might be able to
find the time immediately, but that is not always possible. Here is another option:

> "Mrs. X., I know it is hard to wait when you really want a cigarette, but
> could you help me out please? Could you please wait ten minutes until I
> finish this?"
> "OK."
> "Thanks."

Mrs. X. still doesn't have her cigarette, but at least someone sympathizes
with the way she feels, and there is also something she can do: she can
agree to help Joe out by waiting. Mrs. X. remembers Joe's request for no
more than two minutes before asking for the cigarette again. Again, she
is thanked for waiting. This goes on for ten minutes until Joe can assist
Mrs. X., as he had promised. She may have been annoyed, but it's less
likely that she was annoyed with Joe, because Joe was on her side.

The second approach did not change the repetitive demands or the
interruptions to Joe's work. Repetitive demands and interruptions are a
fact of life when dealing with Alzheimer's disease. It did, however, avoid
a negative interchange. Acrimony and interpersonal distress are not an
inevitable fact of life. We cannot hope to eliminate all challenging or
stressful situations, but we can acknowledge the other person's distress,
validate his position, and bring him around to facing a problem with us
instead of against us. In this way, we can avoid the animosity that is
usually the most painful aspect of any interpersonal altercation.

Some might question the likelihood of Mrs. X.'s accepting the second approach so easily. In fact, it is more likely than we might think. A
cognitively impaired person usually takes her cues from the environment. Approached politely, she is likely to respond politely, because
among most older persons the habitual response to a polite request is a
gracious assent. This strategy takes advantage of established patterns of
behavior. But things do not always work, and no approach is foolproof.
One caregiver tried the "Would you please help me out?" tactic with her
very angry aunt, whose immediate retort was, "Of course, that is all that
you ever think of, yourself. Why should I help you out? Where is my
cigarette?" The caregiver answered simply and calmly, "I'm sorry that
you're upset, Auntie. I'll be back in ten minutes." There are some situa-

tions that are best walked away from. (See Chapter 6 for more discussion of managing and responding to difficult behavior.) However, in most cases we can, by taking control of the situation, keep it in a positive vein and so prevent it from deteriorating into an argument—an argument that a caregiver can never really win.

Another important aspect of nurturing the relationship lies in maintaining a dialogue between the person and yourself. This may take a great deal of courage, especially for family members when they are talking about the person's illness and the difficulties he is experiencing. Ideally, such communication will have started from the first indication of trouble and will go on throughout the course of the person's illness. A particularly difficult decision is whether or not to tell the person that he has Alzheimer's disease. In making this judgment, it is often wise for a family to seek professional counseling.

Although it is a difficult step to take, it is generally much simpler for everyone if the person is told that he has some kind of illness that is affecting his memory and making it difficult for him to continue his affairs as he used to. This takes the pressure off him to try to perform as well as he used to, or to hide the fact that he no longer can. It also gives the caregiver a good hook on which to hang explanations for events that may result from the memory loss. For example, if the person has come to accept reference to his "memory problem," it is much easier to explain the loss of an item that he thinks has been stolen. The explanation may go something like this: "Dad, I think I know what happened to your wallet. I know that it is very important to you and that you always put it in a safe place. That is a smart thing to do. But I wonder if you didn't put it away and now, because of your memory problem, you can't remember where you put it. Do you think that may have happened?" This approach lays blame on the memory and not on the person. It also gives him a way to save face; if he still feels defensive, he can always say no. Then his son can drop the subject, agree with him that it is terrible when things are missing (avoiding any support to the notion that the wallet was stolen), and change the subject. If a dialogue about memory problems has already been established, it is more likely that the person will say "maybe" and then even agree to help in the search for the wallet.

This candor, as difficult as it may seem at the start, pays dividends. It enables the caregiver to continue letting the person know that his difficulty is understood and there is someone here who will help him. It facilitates trust, reduces the person's feeling of having to cover up or defend himself, and helps build a partnership.

Develop an Awareness of Communication Deficits

An awareness of communication deficits involves our understanding the functional and behavioral effects of cognitive impairment in general and, specifically, the nature of the language deficit. Without that understanding, the caregiver relies on gut reactions that may not always be logical or appropriate, and often only add to everyone's frustration. For example, when someone is not understanding us we raise our voice, somehow believing that the increased volume will make things clear. At other times we let our emotions get in the way, and launch into lengthy explanations that the person is unlikely to understand.

Our emotions can also lead us to faulty assumptions. Because we tend to judge people by their capacity to use and understand language, we might assume that a person who is saying things that don't make sense to us is hopelessly confused and doesn't know what he is talking about. Such an assumption undermines trust and respect. It can also jeopardize an existing relationship and hamper the formation of a new one. If a person does not respond appropriately to what we are saying, we assume that he does not understand and is, therefore, unlikely to understand anything. Once again, the relationship is jeopardized by this way of thinking. We have to know what happens to a person's ability to use language in terms of the characteristic disturbances associated with Alzheimer's disease. Then we can make the necessary accommodations to the way we express and receive information. Knowledge of the problem and the application of appropriate strategies give the caregiver control over the situation, help avoid frustration, and provide the tools with which to build and maintain a relationship.

Technical Aspects of Coping with Language Deficit

Speech and Language

The differences between speech and language, and between receptive language and expressive language, need to be clarified. *Speech* is the ability to articulate words, whereas *language* is the ability to conceive the words that will accurately express a thought. Speech is usually unimpaired in persons in the early and middle stages of the illness. It becomes impaired when Parkensonian symptoms accompany Alzheimer's disease or when the person's speech musculature is in some way affected. The person's ability to articulate clearly often deceives caregivers into thinking that there is no intrinsic communication problem, when in fact severe problems may exist. The problem is with language. Even though the person may be saying words well, the words that he uses may not be accurately expressing his thoughts or feelings. He may also have difficulty recognizing words, unraveling long sentences, and keeping track of conversations.

Expressive Language

Expressive language refers to the ability to make oneself understood, whereas *receptive language* refers to the ability to understand. Expressive language problems present themselves in a variety of ways. The person may lose the ability to find the right words to express a thought, or may have difficulty putting a sentence into the correct grammatical order to express it clearly. He may misuse words, substituting words of similar meaning or sound for the intended words, such as "mother" for "daughter" or "wife," or "mouse" for "house." Such errors are called *paraphasic errors*. He may also use *circumlocution,* substituting elaborate descriptive phrases for a single word in an effort to express the thought. "The round color juice thing" might mean "orange." Sometimes the person will revert to the vocabulary and jargon of his former occupation. Whenever she had had enough and wished to be left alone, one lady would very nicely but firmly tell her care provider, "Please go to the next wicket. This station is closed." I do not think that she really believed that she was back in the bank where she had worked for forty years; rather, she was just telling us that she had had enough and wanted to be left alone. In any event, she was satisfied when people just backed off and let her be for a while. On the one occasion when an uninformed attendant responded by trying to orient her to the reality of her retirement from the bank over twenty years ago, she became indignant, quite disoriented, and very upset. Accommodating her as though she had clearly asked for some time out, which in fact she had done, proved to be the most effective response.

As language becomes more and more impaired, it may eventually become a garble of words or near-words that we call a "word salad." On the other hand, the person may be left with only a few repetitive words or phrases with which he tries to express everything. Then the caregiver must rely on understanding the context in which the person is trying to express himself, the person's tone of voice or facial expression, and skill in narrowing the subject down through well-informed guesses.

One gentleman, during an Armistice Day discussion, continued to repeat, "Over the hump, over the hump." No one knew what he meant. The next day the activity director found out from the gentleman's wife where he had seen action during the war. Then she went to the library and asked the librarian to look up for her "over the hump." What could that mean for a Canadian soldier in World War II in Burma? Librarians are generally good resources. They love research, especially a challenge that is also a good puzzle. This librarian came through. The gentleman had been among the Canadian engineers who built the road over the Himalayas that later was known as the "Road to Mandalay." It had been a terrible campaign with horrible conditions and heavy casualties. The librarian provided the activity director with several books of pictures. The gentleman recognized all the pictures and the names of the officers mentioned. He wept at the memory of fallen comrades. When the activity director sympathized with him, saying, "That must have been terrible," he raised his chin and proudly uttered, "No, we won!"

Once again, the responsibility for understanding lies with the caregiver. Our understanding is maximized if we have some insight into the person's pattern of expression and experience.

Questions to Ask to Gain a Better Understanding

Does the person use circumlocutions, nonexistent words (neologisms), or not quite accurate words (paraphasia) to express his thoughts? We can learn his "vocabulary" and so understand him better.

Is there a significant discrepancy between the patient's output when he is speaking spontaneously and when he is replying to questions? The former is usually more fluent and expansive, while the latter may be sparse and labored. Sometimes care providers think that the person is manipulating the conversation when he evades the questions of others and disregards or changes the topic. He is actually seeking his own comfort level by turning to a topic whose words he can say more easily.

Anyone who has learned a new language as an adult will recall the difference between having the freedom to say anything that comes to mind and the restrictions of having to discuss a given topic. In the first instance we can stay within the bounds of our accessible vocabulary. In the second, we desperately search for words and struggle with awkward phrasing trying to get our ideas across.

Is automatic speech, nursery rhymes, counting, and so on, easier than conversational speech? Persons with even very impaired language will sometimes surprise us with a perfect exchange of social niceties or long, accurate recitations of poetry that leave the caregivers wondering how impaired they really are. Family members sometimes suspect that the person may be exaggerating the disability or not really trying. The reality usually is that the person is trying harder than anyone can know. Nursery rhymes, counting, and other habitual bits of language are part of the hardwired system called *overlearned behaviors* that usually remain accessible to even very impaired persons. These patterns are triggered by specific stimuli. They become an automatic reaction which the person does not have to think about or plan, and over which he may even have little control. Things work well when the right trigger facilitates the right reaction at the right time. Word games such as "finish the proverb" or "famous last names" take advantage of this phenomenon and, therefore, usually work very well. Care providers can learn which situations trigger appropriate automatic language reactions and use them more often.

Are emotional utterances and ejaculations preserved when formal speech is defective? Sometimes, especially in a very emotional situation, the person will spew forth a string of swear words that are entirely out of character and very distressing to the family. There are some cases in which it is a cognitively impaired person's loss of judgment and ability to inhibit impulses that leads him to use inappropriate language. Among persons with severe language problems, however, it appears that emotional language and swear words remain the most accessible vocabulary and come out under conditions of stress or excitement. The choice of words is usually not within the person's control, so reprimands or suggestions that he curb his tongue will do little but upset or confuse him. It is best to react to the emotion that the person is expressing, be it anger, pleasure, or whatever, and ignore the words with which he expresses it.

Things to Do to Facilitate Understanding

■ Arm yourself with information. If you are a family member, search your own memory. If you are a professional caregiver, contact family and friends and get the person's history. Go to the library and find out about what was going on during those years so you can place the person's life into a historical context.

■ Read nonverbal language. Facial expressions and gestures may be more revealing than words.

■ Avoid efforts to make the person say the right word. This is not a teaching session. If you are sure of the word that the person is trying to say, say it for him. Most people will be relieved to be let off the hook. If you are not sure, however, your wild guesses may confuse and frustrate the person. Try to narrow the subject down by asking yes or no questions.

■ Put what the person is saying into a context based on your knowledge of what is going on and the language errors this person most frequently makes. Common substitutions are "mother" for "wife" and "last year" for "yesterday." If you know that the person is making the error, make the substitution in your own mind and let him continue.

■ Be aware of your own frustration and back off whenever you start to feel that the situation is futile. But do so with sensitivity, allowing the person to save face.

■ Avoid the temptation to dismiss garbled language or jargon as evidence that the person is "totally confused." Also resist assuming intact language function on the basis of good automatic or spontaneous speech.

■ In everything that you do, strive to reinforce the person's self-esteem and trust. As we have already noted, a person's reactions are dictated by his internal state. If that is a state of trust and comfort, his reactions are more likely to be trusting and comfortable.

■ Find or at least acknowledge meaning in everything that the person says and does.

■ Identify and use the person's remaining skills. Sometimes the most useful skills are overlooked or masked by the dementia. The ability to be polite is one example.

Receptive Language

The other side of language is understanding. A variety of problems can contribute to a person's inability to understand what is being said to him. But even when a person's ability to express himself is very impaired, he may retain some understanding. Here are some questions that may be helpful in determining how much and what kind of understanding remains.

■ Can he point out a specific object when presented with a selection?
■ Can he indicate a response to simple yes or no questions?
■ Can he follow simple orders on request (e.g., pick up an object, clap his hands)?
■ Does he give you the feeling that he understands but can't let you know? Sometimes, as unscientific as it may seem, such intuitive feelings about a person are a valuable measure.

Impediments to Understanding

Lack of Context. In the early stages of the illness, a person who still expresses himself quite well may sometimes have difficulty understanding a statement or question, or picking up the thread of a conversation if the context is not clear. The person may misunderstand references to future or past events, or hypothetical situations. This failure to understand may be evident only as a rise in tension or irritability as he tries to cope and sustain the pretense of understanding.

Inability to Recognize Specific Words. The person with impaired language often ceases to recognize certain words and cannot apply meaning to them when they are spoken to him. Sometimes it will help if the speaker uses a synonym or explains the word in question. The caregiver should take note of the words that create problems and the synonyms or explanations that were understood, and share this information with others who come into contact with the person. In cases where this is a recurrent problem, a lexicon of "words that are well understood" that can be used by everyone in contact with the person can be a very helpful tool. When language function is more impaired, the speaker may have to rely more on nonverbal cues, such as gestures, drawings, or the actual presence of the objects being referred to.

Limited Attention and Distractibility. Difficulty with attention challenges all aspects of function. Understanding language, especially conversational language, demands sustained attention. When a person's ability to focus attention and resist distractions is already compromised, frequent changes of topics in conversation and an environment full of unrelated information can totally undo any remaining ability to understand. Our world is full of extraneous sounds and movement that we filter out without being aware of it. Consequently, we usually do not even notice distractions that acutely interfere with the cognitively impaired person's ability to attend to and, therefore, understand what is said to him.

Inability to Retain Multiple Bits of Information That Constitute the Complex Message. Most of what we say consists of several bits of information that constitute one message. A person with short-term memory impairment may be able to remember only one or two of these bits and, consequently, will not be able to make sense of a complex, multiple-component message. He may be so busy trying to remember the first bit that all that follows goes unnoticed. Or each subsequent bit knocks the preceding information out of his memory, resulting in his remembering only the last bit of whatever message is spoken.

How to Help

- Minimize dependence on spoken language for communication.
- Remain sensitive to the fact that, although the person may not understand your words, he retains the ability to read your body language, your mood, and your sincerity.
- Support what you say with appropriate gestures. For example, if you want the person to sit down, point to a specific chair as you ask him to sit.
- Use short, simple phrases, addressing one topic at a time.
- Conduct important conversations in a place that is free from distractions.
- Do not assume that the person whose expressive ability is impaired is unable to understand what is being said around him.

Written Language

One of the most common devices caregivers use to help a person cope with failing memory is written cues and notes. However, what was once very effective can become a source of frustration when the person loses the ability to comprehend written language. One way to find out is by objective observation. Can the person follow a simple written instruction, such as "clap your hands"? Even though the patient may be able to read aloud, he may not understand what he is reading. If that becomes the case, reliance on written notices or signs for orientation or reminders should be discontinued.

Some General and Practical Approaches to Communication

- Always approach the cognitively impaired person in an open, friendly, and gentle manner, even if the situation demands urgency or has caused you to be upset. If you are tense and anguished, the person will also become tense and anguished.
- Always address the person by name at the beginning of your statement to make sure that you have his attention.
- Make sure that you give your full attention to the conversation or task at hand. Your attentive energy will help keep the person focused. If, on the other hand, you are distracted or preoccupied, the person will feel that also and will find it even more difficult to stay with the subject.
- Unless the person gives you positive evidence that he remembers

you and has placed you in the correct context, do not assume that he recognizes you. Unless you know, it is best to introduce yourself and include some orientation cues each time you approach the person. In addition to stating your name, you might, for example, mention your relation to him, the purpose of your visit, and how long since you've last seen him. However, keep the information pertinent and avoid long-winded explanations.

- Speak slowly, but do not "speak down" to the person.
- Use physical expressions of caring, such as gentle touching or holding hands, but make sure that you first have the person's permission to intrude into their personal space. Some people are private and defensive of their personal space and will take offense if approached abruptly.
- If the person is reacting negatively or becoming upset, avoid arguing and attempts to reason. Instead, acknowledge the feelings you think the person is expressing and calmly take him to a comfortable place or activity to calm him down. It is important that the person perceive you as a source of comfort and security, not an adversary. If the things you try are not working, calmly take the person to someone else whom the person may perceive as a protector. This approach requires teamwork and needs to be taught to staff as part of their in-service training.

Once you have discovered an approach, phrase, or insight that works well, note it exactly, share it with other caregivers, and use it consistently. Consistency is one of the most effective tools in caring for persons with Alzheimer's disease. Sometimes we may think that we are being consistent, but actually we are introducing subtle differences into our phrases or instructions. We may believe that these changes clarify and elaborate the sense of what we are saying, but in most cases they are merely confusing. For example, we might think that "soon," "in a little while," "in less than five minutes," and "in a bit" all mean the same thing. To us they may, but to a person whose understanding is already challenged, each phrase is a new bit of information that needs to be newly interpreted.

Another barrier to communication is fear: our fear of hurting the person, fear of losing control over the situation, or fear of generating uncomfortable emotions in the person. All these fears are manifested in the dilemma of whether or not to tell the person about things that will cause sadness or grief, such as the death or illness of a loved one. Everyone is familiar with "the case of the forgetful mourner." Whenever a memory-impaired person asks about a loved one who is deceased, the caregiver must choose whether to tell him the truth, with the risk of shocking him and restarting again the painful mourning process, or to shield him by devising some other kind of explanation. The difficulty is that we never know for sure whether he is asking for information or seeking confirmation of something that he already knows or suspects. Another problem is that any duplicity we have arranged to avoid answering the question must eventually be exposed. Can you imagine your own confusion and loss of trust if you thought that you were the object of a conspiracy? Consider also the lack of respect for the person that such an approach implies, as well as the isolation that it creates. See Chapter 6 for more discussion of this problem.

Communication is much more than an exchange of information. It also involves personal contact, and words are not the only way in which such contact is made. In fact, even among fully articulate people, you sometimes find that even after a million words have been exchanged, there has been no real connection, no real communication. Yet at other times a glance, a touch of the hand, or a smile creates such a connection between two people that words are superfluous. True communication is not mere physical proximity or the exchange of information or ideas. There is something else: a personal presence. When words are no longer understood, we can make our presence felt through touch, tone of voice, songs, facial expressions, holding and rocking or swinging hands, cooing and "loving" sounds, or even just silent attention. This is how we create the connection that is true communication.

A question frequently asked of those who work with persons who have Alzheimer's disease is, "Don't you find it exhausting to try to communicate with a person who has so much trouble speaking and understanding?" The words of de Castillejo are an eloquent response to that question: "We are only exhausted when talking to other people if we do not meet them, when one or both of us are hiding behind screens. On the rare occasions when we are fortunate enough to meet someone, there is no question of fatigue. Both are refreshed, for something has happened. It is as though a door had opened, and life suddenly takes on new meaning" (De Castillejo 1974, 11).

10

Alzheimer's Disease and the Home: Issues in Environmental Design

Said Dorothy, upon returning from Oz, "There's no place like home!" Indeed, no place presents so many variables in design, history, significance, and emotional attachments. There is no standard description for a home. It may be a lifelong habitation or a new apartment. It may be a busy home where three generations live or it may be a bachelor suite for one. The home is usually thought of positively, as a place that represents security and comfort and that positively reflects significant roles from a person's past and facilitates the use of retained abilities. Unfortunately, to some cognitively impaired persons the familiar setting may be a persistent reminder of frustration and lost skills, provoking depression or stimulating activities that are no longer appropriate or even safe. This variability makes generalizations about environmental design for the homes of people with Alzheimer's disease particularly challenging.

Any discussion of environmental design for housing persons with Alzheimer's disease must consider three basic areas: factors that will aid in preserving their function for as long as possible, those that will affect their safety, and those that will promote emotional well-being. In addition, when considering the domestic environment, the needs of caregivers must receive attention. This discussion is, therefore, divided into four basic sections: preservation of function, safety, emotional well-being, and caregiver needs.

Preserving Function

Excess disability is a term that describes a degree of functional decline that cannot be attributed solely to the person's level of organic impairment (Brody et al. 1971). It is believed to be due partly to the impaired person's inability to extract meaningful information from the environment and, consequently, to act in a constructive and coherent manner (Haugen 1985). It follows, then, that the environment can have a significant influence on preserving the individual's functional ability. A facili-

148

tating environment promotes an optimal level of function in the individual. It helps the person take full advantage of his retained abilities by accommodating for his deficits and by providing an outlet for his individual needs.

Among the abilities most commonly retained by persons with Alzheimer's disease are old, overlearned patterns of movement. Objects in the environment that provoke these old patterns of behavior will be most facilitating: for example, a clock with hands instead of a digital model, a sink of soapy water instead of a dishwasher, a rotary phone instead of a touch-tone model.

Just as familiar articles facilitate function, innovative or modern objects can disable skills. There is no telling how often modern, one-handed faucets, touch-tone phones, and security intercom systems in apartment lobbies have inhibited the independent function of persons who, despite mild and moderate impairment, had been managing adequately with the old, conventional items.

Another way in which the environment can facilitate function is by accommodating for the person's deficits. Many of the common errors and distressing behaviors exhibited by the person with Alzheimer's disease, such as urinating in inappropriate places or misusing objects, result from impaired perception and judgment. The best response to such problems is to simplify the environment and remove the confusing or misguiding cues. A facilitating environment will diminish the potential for such errors and accidents by providing only the articles appropriate for a specific task.

A third characteristic of the facilitating environment is the provision of an outlet for the individual's special needs, in particular, the need to move about, the need to discharge strong emotions, and the need for sensory stimulation. These needs seem to be behind much of the perplexing or challenging behavior that persons with Alzheimer's disease exhibit. Pacing and wandering is often a way of dissipating excess energy and getting sensory feedback from joint and muscle movements. Physical movement that feels good can be facilitated by the use of a stationary bicycle, a treadmill, or a rocking chair. Caregivers have reported on the usefulness of such equipment in the home (Gilleard et al. 1984).

The venting of emotions such as anger and frustration is a universal need. The person with Alzheimer's disease is often dependent on nonverbal means of expression and is unable to identify appropriate means for satisfying this need. A facilitating environment makes such opportunities available and obvious. Hitting a punching bag, pounding dough, and digging in a garden have been suggested as possible ways of venting strong emotions in a socially acceptable way (Hiatt 1987).

The need for sensory stimulation has already been mentioned, but cannot be overemphasized. Tactile stimulation has been repeatedly identified in the literature as an important source of sensory input. Unfortunately, as a person becomes more impaired and in greater need of this basic form of stimulation, the surrounding textures of clothing, upholstery, wood, and so on, tend to be replaced with smooth, easily cleaned surfaces that lack those sensual qualities. When a person is offered sensory materials to handle, it is essential that the materials be appropriate to that person's social status, and that anything that could be perceived as infantalizing be scrupulously avoided (Zgola 1990).

Safety

Impaired memory, faulty judgment, and undirected energy make the person with Alzheimer's disease prone to dangerous behavior. The home that is designed to support a normal community lifestyle is full of potential hazards. Electrical and gas appliances, tools, and household chemicals may trigger familiar but dangerous patterns of behavior for a person who no longer has the judgment to act safely.

Along with sleep disturbances that cause nighttime rousing (Sanford 1975), the constant vigilance needed to prevent mishaps and dangerous wandering is identified as the greatest source of caregiver stress (Gilleard et al. 1982). Long-term care facilities cope by providing specially designed areas with clear sightlines and surveillance by around-the-clock staff. Wandering is controlled by locking the exits or monitoring them with electronic alarms. Because the facility is dedicated solely to the safe maintenance and comfort of residents, it is possible to keep potentially dangerous materials and equipment permanently stowed away.

Although some of these alternatives are available to the caregiver at home and usually help create a safer environment, they may cause their own problems. Exits can be secured with hidden or complicated locks, dangerous appliances can be disconnected or otherwise disabled, and hazardous objects can be stored. But when such measures interfere with an impaired person's entrenched behavior patterns, they can provoke angry outbursts. Even a simple, commonly used solution such as a hidden lock can cause an incident when the person, despite his inability to open the new lock, remembers that the door always used to open and should now. Confronted with a desire to go out and a door that will not open, he may respond with anger and frustration; the solution has become yet another problem. A stove that no longer works because the fuses have been removed for safety's sake, may prompt a lady to persist in calling the landlord or to go out in pursuit of help. People have been known to turn an entire house upside down looking for a treasured object that had been removed for safekeeping.

This phenomenon has been termed "agenda behavior" and is described as behavior that is a response to a physical, social, or emotional need (Rader et al. 1985). Efforts to thwart such behavior without offering an alternative often result in an intensification of the behavior or in an even more dangerous effort to overcome the obstacle. A gate across the top of a staircase can be even more dangerous than the open stairs; the person who is accustomed to negotiating the stairs might slip and fall, but he is far more likely to have a serious accident attempting to climb over a gate in an effort to get downstairs. The gate, rather than preventing an accident, could trigger a very dangerous act. The lady who attempts to pry open a locked door with a kitchen knife may cause more damage and place herself in greater jeopardy than if she had merely gone outside.

When a door is locked or any other object is made inaccessible, it is often useful to disguise it as well, so that it no longer acts as a stimulus. It also helps to provide an obvious and equally interesting alternative. If a thermostat cover is installed to prevent a person from adjusting the temperature, it would help to have the cover match the color of the wall. If one closet is barred, another to which the person has free access should be obviously available.

Sometimes it may be easier to install a simple monitoring device such as a bell that will inform the caregiver of the person's movements without actually interfering with them. In many cases a squeaky door or a creaking floorboard makes a good monitor. Any device that will alert the caregiver that the person is "on the move" will reduce the stress of constant vigilance. Some families find that a simple intercom system, such as is used to monitor a child's room, is enough to give them peace of mind. Complex locks that are obviously positioned may slow the person in his attempts to go out without frustrating him unduly, and still give the caregivers enough time to be alerted to his movements and to divert or accompany him.

Potentially dangerous behavior is not limited to persons with dementing illnesses. We all have some risky habits, such as climbing on unstable stools to reach heights, or using a soapdish or towel rack as a handhold for getting up from the bathtub. We have also all been guilty of oversights that have or could have had disastrous consequences. A cognitively impaired person continues to take risks as part of his long-standing, habitual patterns of behavior, but unlike a healthy person is usually incapable of either checking a dangerous act before a mishap occurs or taking quick action to limit the damage when an accident does happen. A person with Alzheimer's disease retains most of these potentially dangerous habits and is even more prone than a healthy person to such blunders as leaving the pot to boil dry or the iron on and sitting on its faceplate. Moreover, because of impaired judgment and problem-solving skills this person is far more vulnerable to the consequences of such acts.

Fortunately, consumer concern for home safety has prompted the design and general availability of many safety devices and appliances with built-in safety features; some examples are smoke detectors, electric kettles and steam irons with automatic shutoffs, and water temperature regulators that can be installed at the faucet while still permitting hot water flow to the laundry and dishwasher. The advantage of such devices is that they limit the amount of danger to which a person with Alzheimer's disease is exposed without interfering with his habitual patterns of behavior and independence.

This same principle should be applied anywhere that alterations to promote safety are made. When a new device is introduced, it should be done so that it fits into the person's habitual patterns of behavior. Grab bars, for example, should replace the old unsafe handholds, even if this means that they are not in the ideal location. Otherwise the person is likely to continue using the unsafe toilet paper holder, towel rack or soapdish and ignore the newly added grab bars.

There are many dangerous items in our homes which we have learned to live with and even ignore. Slippery throw rugs and loose carpet edges can cause a fall. Low coffee tables can cause a person to trip or bump a shin. Not only is a person with Alzheimer's disease more vulnerable to such accidents, but his ability to cope with injury and its resulting hospitalization or restriction of movement is lower. Injuries often have the unfortunate effect of accelerating functional decline in a cognitively impaired person.

In summary, the solution is not solely to limit the person's access to potentially dangerous areas or to remove or deactivate appliances and secure hazardous substances. The person's need to be active must also be served by providing safe and meaningful activities and the materials with which to pursue them (Zgola 1987).

Emotional Well-Being

The need for meaningful stimulation and occupation is universal. Many authors discuss the cognitively impaired person's need for adequate sensory stimulation (Woods and Britton 1985; Paire and Karney 1984). Coons and Weaverdyck (1986) observed behavioral changes in persons who were provided with significant activity. The importance of self-directed activity and causation is pointed out by Keilhoffner (1983). But perhaps the most poignant comment on the importance of having something meaningful to do comes from A. B. Lerner's documentation of some of his cognitively impaired wife's early morning comments: "I would rather be dead than what I am doing here because I am not doing anything. . . . The worst thing is not having anything to do. I can't take it" (Lerner 1984).

A special place in the home, set aside for the person's habitual activities, can provide both respite for the caregiver and meaningful activity for the person. One gentleman "accident-proofed" his wife's sewing room by removing all valuable items that could be damaged or destroyed by her sometimes misguided efforts to mend, and provided her with items of clothing that could be safely snipped and sewed. He bought an iron that automatically shuts off when placed faceplate down or is left standing for a set period of time. For some time, she continued to use the sewing machine skillfully, but when she began to confuse the controls her husband removed it with the explanation that it needed repair, and thereafter she was limited to hand-sewing. For several hours each day she puttered in her sewing room, surrounded by the things that had given her comfort and self-esteem in the past. A similar arrangement could be made in a workshop, a potting shed, or a garden when the objective is redirected from the product of the work to the person's pleasure in doing it.

Impaired memory, judgment, and problem-solving abilities make a person with Alzheimer's disease vulnerable to the stresses of disorientation and catastrophic reactions (Mace and Rabins 1981). The more impaired the individual, the more dependent she will be on a supportive physical environment to maintain emotional stability (Lawton 1984). A supportive environment will promote orientation and provide security, and will also prompt memory and recollection. Any mechanisms that improve orientation and clarity of perception will contribute to the individual's sense of security, and therefore to her emotional well-being. Lighting is one way to enhance perception. More light should be available in places where the person is expected to concentrate or engage in activities such as grooming, dressing, or leisure pursuits that require focus. Lighting can also be adjusted to aid the person finding her way by dimming the light in the corridor and brightening it at the destination (Lawton 1984). Marking edges of stairs with contrasting tape assists the person in judging depth. It has been suggested that colored tape around the edge of a bathtub will offer extra cues regarding its shape and depth.

Labeling doors and objects in the home and posting written instructions and reminders may sometimes be useful. In the author's experience, such labeling is most helpful to facilitate language in early-stage persons who have word-finding difficulties, or to orient mildly impaired persons to a new home. Written instructions are useful in supporting the functional abilities of mildly impaired individuals, but by the time a person has become disoriented to the location of specific rooms or objects in their habitual home, labels usually do little to assist orientation and written reminders may even add to the confusion. A better way to assist orientation at that time is to leave doors to important rooms, such as the bedroom and bathroom, opened. The person will be less likely to rummage for things if the doors of frequently used closets and cupboards are left opened or even removed altogether. Multisensory stimulation is another aid to orientation. The more senses a particular situation stimulates, the more clearly that situation will be perceived (Snyder 1978). Specific sounds, odors, textures, colors, and movements are habitually associated with specific places and activities. These sensations, provided that they are consistent with one another and are not overwhelming, enhance the person's orientation to a situation, or promote behavior that is appropriate. Features that evoke such sensations are being incorporated into new institutional designs, but they already exist in wonderful variety within the home. The kitchen usually smells and sounds like someone is cooking. Laundry day smells of bleach and detergent. The living room may smell of furniture polish and be a place for rocking and listening to music.

Unfortunately, as a person with Alzheimer's disease becomes more impaired, safety and physical care gradually take precedence, in the caregiver's mind, over these trappings of everyday life. Rooms are gradually stripped of breakable or dangerous items, and the caregiver's diminished energy limits the amount of "nonessential" activity that goes on in the home. There is a danger that the person's environment will be depleted of those essential sights, smells, activities, and sounds that promote awareness and orientation. An effective use of community home support services is to provide home-based respite that will free a caregiver to resume some of those activities that used to contribute to and enhance that homelike atmosphere (Zgola 1988).

Just as some stimuli contribute to orientation, other objects and stimuli contribute to disorientation by provoking misperceptions or distractions. Shiny and reflective surfaces, glare, and shadows may distort visual perception. Shiny floors look wet and interfere with perception of distance. Mirrors distress persons who no longer recognize their own reflections by creating the illusion that other people are in the room. Windows produce the same effect at night unless drapes or blinds are pulled. Shadows can create illusions of objects, spaces, or movement. Background noise can interfere with hearing and distort auditory perception. Finally, multiple stimuli such as conflicting radio and television, multiple conversations, and extraneous movements draw the person's attention in different directions and are likely to be confusing and distressing. Such distractions should, therefore, be eliminated whenever possible.

In the home of a person with Alzheimer's disease, one always draws a fine line between making alterations to promote safety and preserving sameness to promote security and orientation (Gnaedinger 1989). As items that are potentially dangerous or upsetting are removed and safety devices are introduced, it is often helpful to bring in safe, comforting articles from the past that represent more stable times. Photographs, tools, handicrafts, keepsakes, and other belongings that are recognized and identified with good memories often help aid orientation and reminiscence. This is especially helpful if the person no longer recognizes the present home and becomes agitated and distressed with the desire to return to an older home or to some vague memory of "home." Familiar objects can help to recapture those old, satisfying experiences (Zgola and Coulter 1988).

The Needs of the Caregiver

The home in which a person with Alzheimer's disease lives must also support the lifestyle needs of the caregiver and other family members. In a recent survey, family caregivers reported that the most needed physical feature in the home was a private place for themselves (Gnaedinger 1989). As the home is gradually modified to accommodate the cognitively impaired person, and as the caregiver's time is almost exclusively devoted to caring for that individual, the need for personal, inviolate space and time increases. This need for privacy and time alone is also reflected in reports of caregivers who cope with the strain by setting up situations in which they can temporarily ignore or distance themselves from the person they are caring for.

When the cognitively impaired person is sharing a family home, the personal effects and privacy of other family members must also be safeguarded. This can sometimes be accomplished by isolating the living quarters of the person and limiting her access to certain areas occupied by other family members. Another alternative is to install locks on private rooms, preventing intrusion. If such arrangements are not possible, there is a danger that conflict and resentments will develop. This may jeopardize family integrity and the support system that is essential in maintaining a person with Alzheimer's disease in the home. In fact, it is often the psychological and social problems related to living with the person, rather than difficulties with physical care, that precipitate placement outside of the home.

Conclusion

Although not all persons with Alzheimer's disease exhibit the same behaviors and vulnerabilities, there are some patterns of disabilities, preserved abilities, and needs that are characteristic. While generalizations are useful, they are made with the understanding that individual characteristics and behaviors must be considered. Not only do individuals vary, but each individual varies from day to day. In the face of a progressive condition, solutions that worked one week may cease to be effective by the next, and problems that were paramount one week may in time dissipate.

It is difficult to limit a discussion of the role of the environment in the care of persons with Alzheimer's disease exclusively to "bricks and mortar" issues. Attitudes, relationships, and programs are so much a part of any environment that they can make up for many physical shortcomings, or negate the positive effects of even the most ideal physical setting. This is true of any residential setting, but is particularly true of the home. Although the caregivers surveyed by Gnaedinger identified some practical physical accommodations that can be made, they all maintained that their greatest needs were for more trained helpers, more education, and, especially, more respite. Physical design issues, therefore, constitute only a part of the picture when it comes to keeping a person with Alzheimer's disease in the home. Programs that provide social and emotional support and respite for the caregiver are essential. Without such support, without relief from the need for constant vigilance, even the most commonly advocated physical adaptations in the home are virtually useless.

11

Programming Activities

There is probably no more valuable tool in the care of persons with Alzheimer's disease than meaningful activity. Used well, it can raise spirits and dispel depression. It can calm restlessness and agitation. It can bring comfort to a person who is distressed. When two people sit down to a task together, they immediately have something in common. Activity programming is not a frill; it is essential, no less important than physical care and nutrition.

Activity programming is not simply keeping people busy after all the instrumental aspects of care have been seen to. It is a total process in which each person is offered the opportunity to live in the manner best suited to him, and to continue doing the things that promote his sense of security, efficacy, membership, and personal value. Such programming must be delivered competently and judiciously by caregivers who understand its value, are knowledgeable about its techniques, and have the training and support to do it well. Just as with any other aspect of care, misguided or inappropriate programming is ineffective at best and at worst can do harm.

This chapter does not offer a listing of possible activities. It describes a process by which caregivers identify, plan, and offer activities that are meaningful and satisfying for the individuals in their care. A list is limited, whereas a process offers an unlimited number of possibilities.

Why Is Activity Important?

"Doing," to most people, is synonymous with being alive. The vast majority of people continue to do things of their choosing until the day they die. The tragedy of Alzheimer's disease is that it removes from a living person the capacity to do things years and years before the body is ready to stop. Let's walk for a moment in the shoes of a person who can no longer "do."

You have spent a lifetime doing so many things—difficult things, amusing things, interesting things, things that you had to get done, things that you wanted to get done. Sometimes there were just so many things to do that you wished they would stop. There were times when people praised you and thanked you for the things you did, and other times when they rebuked you. You remember slaving over a difficult task and then standing back to look at a job well done. The best thing of all, probably, was kicking back and relaxing because you knew that you'd earned the rest.

Now you still have the desire and the energy to do things, but they just do not work for you any more. You start something and things go wrong. Sometimes people ask you to do something and you just do not know how to start. They say you are getting lazy. You just feel left out, controlling nothing, effecting nothing, and needed by no one.

Small changes started some time ago. You stopped going to the club one winter because the sidewalk was too icy. Then the garden became too difficult, so they had someone in to tend it for you. You kept a flower box on the balcony for a while and that was nice. It helped you get over the fact that the young lad was not keeping the perennial beds the way you used to. They suggested that you sell your car. It would be so much easier to have your groceries delivered, and you didn't really go anywhere except to the doctor. You could always get a volunteer driver for that. Then the homemaker started to come more often because your laundry wasn't getting done often enough. That was OK. Actually, it was quite pleasant because she would let you help take it off the line and fold it, and that smelled so nice and reminded you of when the kids were little. There was so much laundry to do then.

She cooked well, too—for a foreigner, that is. But when they started saying how good *her* cookies were, that was a bit too much. Didn't they remember *your* shortbread? If she had at least used your recipes or asked you for some advice so that you could have had just a little hand in things, it wouldn't seem as though you had lost so much ground. You started to resent her and told them that you didn't like her, figured she was breaking the china and maybe even stealing from the grocery money. They brought in a new one. She didn't want to hang out the wash so she took it to the laundromat and brought it back all folded. That left nothing much for you to do with that.

When they noticed that you weren't doing much of anything anymore, and maybe you had complained about it once or twice, they sent you to a day program. Everyone there was very nice. They were quite efficient, did everything to make sure you would have fun, games, crafts, bus trips. They were so good at their jobs that sometimes you felt like a fifth wheel. It was as though you were at a perpetual birthday party. Was it that they thought you couldn't do much? You wondered if they knew that you had been the first woman school principal in the district. Would they have asked you to help more often if they had had any idea just how competent you could be? But you are no fool, after all. How can you complain about having not enough work and too much fun? But somehow something was missing in that place. Maybe you were just saying "thank you" so often and hearing it said to you so seldom that you started wondering what the point was of your being around.

Then at home someone must have told the homemaker about your fall in the bathtub, because she started to insist on watching you take your shower. "My God," you shouted. "Let me do at least that much for myself. What will you want to do next? Feed me?!" They said that you were over-reacting. That it was really nothing and you had to expect such things at your age. There was a second fall and then they made sure that she gave you your bath. Oh, the indignity! At least she took the time to scrub your back; that was something that you had really never been able to do for yourself, and that made the whole thing tolerable.

Altogether, though, you are still better off than your neighbor, Nora, who is at the home. At least you can get up any time you want, except on day program days. You hear that they get Nora up and dressed by eight o'clock every day. "Preserve me from that," you think. At least you still have your own fridge that you can go to any time you want, as long as the homemaker remembers to buy your favorite snacks. You still have your apartment. You have the things that you and your husband collected and that remind you of the life you spent together.

What would it be like to lose that too, the way Nora has? Is she allowed to decide anything for herself? you wonder. Do they dress her? Feed her? Does she have to hand over her dentures for them to clean? Do they give her toys to keep her busy the way they would with a child? What if that ever happened to you?

With these things going through your mind, think of how you would feel: lost, useless, afraid, angry, worthless, dependent, out of control, like a nobody, or sad.

What have you lost or are you in danger of losing? Control, connection with others, efficacy, usefulness, value, identity, and fun. What do you need? To do something. You need a program of activities and life experiences that will restore your sense of yourself as a valued, responsible, loved, and loving individual. This is the aim of responsible and responsive activity programming.

Because each person is unique, programming must be individually planned. Because a person's needs are met by doing the whole range of things that make up his life, the program must draw from the full spectrum of daily activities, as well as special events. Because a person with Alzheimer's disease faces a real and pervasive disability, the program must be presented in a way that compensates for his disability and lets him make full use of his remaining skills.

A Special Responsibility

A special responsibility in programming for persons with Alzheimer's disease arises because they are not only physically dependent but also emotionally dependent. Therefore, the activity that is offered, the way it is offered, and the outcome of the activity all have a very direct influence on how the person feels about himself and those who care for him. If the activity seems childish, or if it is too difficult, if the product does not meet the person's standards, he has no way to account for these impressions, but simply experiences humiliation, frustration, and failure.

The traditional methods of activity programming no longer work. Set programs that require the participants' initiative and insightful cooperation do not serve this population. Persons with dementia rarely consult the activity schedule, even less often choose activities from the board, and hardly ever show up on their own at the activities for which they have been designated. When the activities staff try to apply the old methods by spending time posting schedules, collecting participants for activities, and trying to keep them there, they have little time left to do what these people really need: to be allowed and helped to do things most resembling what they would be doing if they had not become ill. This population needs activities that come to them, engage them directly and spontaneously, and fit into their normal routine of life, not a schedule. Seen from this perspective, activity programming becomes a model of care.

Characteristics of Programming

In dementia care, we can talk about therapeutic activity programming. It will not reverse the condition, but it will lift the effects of sensory deprivation, social withdrawal, and functional decline and break the cycle that leads to excess disability.

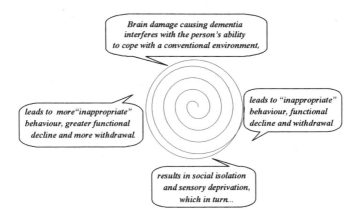

The tragic spiral of functional decline

Individually planned activities and meaningful relationships offer a supportive environment and promote success. Success encourages the person to remain active and make full use of his remaining abilities. A frequent consequence of such well-planned and executed programs is that participants exceed the caregivers' expectations. They demonstrate strengths and resources that were not previously evident.

Teamwork is a concept that must be taken seriously. Activity programming with this broad perspective cannot be the responsibility of any one person or department. Although the activity professional may be the prime mover and coordinator, everyone who comes into contact with the resident or participant must also appreciate their responsibility. Here is a wonderful opportunity and challenge for the various disciplines involved with the person to work as a real team. The team includes nursing and activities, housekeeping, dietary, and whatever other staff directly or indirectly have a hand in creating the resident's environment. This means regular team conferences, consistent communication, and a stated commitment from everyone. There must also be a means of involving and sharing information with families, visitors, and volunteers. A well-articulated program must be understood by and accessible to everyone.

This kind of programming not only serves the best interests of the participants but also makes activities a rewarding experience for all the staff members involved. By thinking things through from basic principles, by knowing what they are doing and why they are doing it, they

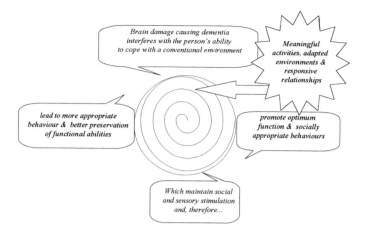

Breaking the tragic spiral of functional decline

have control. They also avoid those frantic searches for something to do that can be such a nightmare. Above all, everyone, both caregivers and participants, has fun.

The Nature of Meaningful Activity

A meaningful activity meets several criteria: it has purpose; it is done voluntarily; it feels good to the participant; it is socially appropriate; and it imparts a sense of success. These same criteria are essential in any activity that is offered to cognitively impaired participants.

Every Activity Must Have an Obvious Purpose

There is nothing that anyone does for no reason at all. No matter how silly or frivolous it may seem, there is a reason for everything we do. The reason may be that the activity simply feels good, or it may be as complex as raising money for a new appliance. Whatever it is, the purpose must be obvious and acceptable to everyone involved.

Many cognitively impaired persons go along with activity programs that are set out for them even though they do not grasp the purpose. They find their own purpose in attending. It may be the socialization, it may be recognition by the staff, or it may just be that there is nothing else to do. Let's think for a moment, then, why we are doing this collage. Perhaps we are looking at the pictures, choosing our favorites, and enjoying good company while we do it. In that case we are looking through magazines and socializing. We could perhaps dispense with the glue, scissors, and construction paper and just have cookies while we look through magazines, talk about the most interesting pictures, and have a good time.

Every Activity Must Be Voluntary

Even though getting the cognitively impaired person involved may require some encouragement, explanation, and modeling, the person must eventually come to the activity willingly. There is no meaning in activities that are forced on a person. Caregivers must be alert to the person who does things just to please the staff. It may be important to this person that she is accepted, but there must be other ways for the person to achieve security. It may also be that there is nothing else to do. Participation should not be a matter of default. Far too often, participants in wheelchairs are simply brought to the program. This is not voluntary and hence not meaningful participation.

Every Activity Must Be Pleasurable

The person who is unable to remember cannot anticipate and, consequently, lives entirely in the here-and-now. In that state, there is no such thing as present pain for future gain. If, for any reason, the activity does not feel good to the person, stop it. Reconsider or redirect, but do not continue. The cues are not only in the verbal messages that participants give. The nonverbal messages are often more accurate. Activity facilitators must always be aware of negative and positive body language during the course of any activity or encounter.

Every Activity Must Be Socially Appropriate

The activity and the product of the activity must be a positive reflection of the person's age and status. There is no harm in doing silly and childish things when everyone knows that they are adults who have just decided to be silly. A cognitively impaired person may not see it the same way. Persevering autonomy and self-esteem are often an ongoing struggle of long standing for this person. An activity that appears childish or silly may threaten an already vulnerable self-image. It can be a devastating blow.

The product that comes out of a program must reflect the competence of the participants, not their disability. Products of high quality do not necessarily require high levels of skill. Any painting done on good-quality paper and properly framed will be a work of art, while a painting done on construction paper and tacked to a board will look like the product of a kindergarten class. Several frames and mats can be purchased to display the residents' work in rotation.

Consideration of the product of a program is a very important aspect of preserving the dignity and social status of program participants, and the respect of the staff. How can staff members consistently relate as adults to participants and residents whose construction paper and crayon art is displayed on the walls with each one's first name written by the coordinator on the bottom? It is also an issue for friends and families. When family members are unable to distinguish Granny's work from that of little Johnny as it hangs on the refrigerator door, it is a tragedy. Moreover, it is absolutely unnecessary.

Cost is not an issue. Good materials and well-thought-out programs pay for themselves, not only in morale but also in dollars. The products can be sold, which builds participants' morale and goes to pay for more good-quality materials. Good materials are often available free. Small scrap pieces of fine wood from a furniture manufacturer, sanded and oiled, make nice cutting boards. Even smaller ones can be used as the base for wall plaques decorated with pressed flowers or decoupage (Zgola 1987). Participants can contribute to such products by doing whatever they are able to do well. It could be sanding, pasting, or applying the many coats of clear finish to create a fine product.

Concrete, durable products are not the most important outcome of an activity. Instead of making plasticine figurines, why not have the same sensory and creative experience with gingerbread dough? When the manual experience is done, we put them in the oven, bake (sterilize) them, create a wonderful fragrance, and serve them, giving the participants the taste and the pleasure of sharing a product that everyone can enjoy and be proud of. A good time in the company of friends yields good feelings, which are the best product possible.

There comes a point when a cognitively impaired person may no longer be aware of the adult or childish nature of the activities offered her. We never really know, but even when all indications suggest that she is not aware, there is a reason to be concerned about the age-appropriateness of the activities offered. The activity in which a person is engaged is a reflection of that person. If she is engaged in something that appears childish, such as cuddling a pink plush toy, for example, the image she projects is that of a poor little old lady who is in her "second childhood," and that is how most people are likely to treat her. If she is holding a beautifully crafted pillow or decorator stuffed animal made of corduroy or velour with lace and brocade trim, she will get the same comfort from holding a soft, warm object on her lap, but the image she projects will be one of a lady who appreciates nice things, and that is how she will most likely be treated.

Every Activity Must Be Failure-Proof

Keeping in mind that any activity should be a positive, affirming experience for the participant, every possible effort must be made to ensure success. Many of the participants have been coping with failure for years before coming to us; it is time that it stopped. The activities that are offered must be within the person's abilities to perform. Little is gained in the way of success and achievement from complex projects that staff members do while participants watch. This is not a meaningful activity, and is at best a waste of time. It may also be a demeaning, perplexing, and defeating experience for the participants. Furthermore, it is absolutely unnecessary. There is a myriad of activities that are utterly failure-proof: sweeping the floor, raking leaves, drying dishes, dusting, offering advice, and supervising someone else in an activity are just a few examples. The point is to see the activity from the participants' perspective, not from that of an observer in the room.

If the activity does fail, the responsibility lies with the caregiver to minimize the negative impact of the experience on the cognitively impaired person. This might mean absorbing the blame, making a joke, or quickly recovering or redirecting the activity so that it works out another way. Any such efforts must be realistic. If the person does associate the failure with her own incompetence, she may just need comfort and an understanding ear. Sometimes it is possible to prepare for the potential failure of an untried project by simply making the objective finding out whether or not it will work. We can find out, for example, whether it is possible to make good muffins in this microwave.

The Scope of Meaningful Activity

The activities that are meaningful will differ from individual to individual. Fortunately the choice of potentially meaningful activities reaches far beyond the structured activities that include art, music, discussion groups, reminiscence, and exercise. A program that limits itself to these activities severely limits the possible range of enjoyable, rewarding, and meaningful activity for its participants and sets itself an almost

The scope of meaningful activity

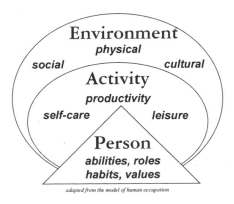

A model-defining activity (adapted from Canadian Association of Occupational Therapists 1991)

unrealizable challenge. How can a set program of groups, crafts, exercise, and outings hope to meet the diversity of interests, needs, and abilities that is present in a group of forty to a hundred persons over seventy years old with various degrees of cognitive impairment? It is impossible. Fortunately, living offers a much wider range of activities than any activity director could conceive. These often overlooked activities include the simple tasks of daily living, caring for oneself, helping others, doing chores, relaxing, thinking, and watching, as well as crafts, discussions, exercise, and entertainments.

To achieve a frame of reference, we can look at a model. Activity can be defined as a person's interaction with the environment. The environment consists of physical, social, and cultural aspects. Activity takes place within three spheres of activity: productivity, self-care, and leisure.

Spheres of Activity

Productivity

Work and work roles are an important aspect of most people's lives and often remain so even after retirement. Most seniors, when asked about the most important thing they have done recently, cite some task or responsibility that they have rendered either to their community or their family. Unfortunately, many persons in care settings are likely to say that they have not done anything important recently. The loss of productivity, the capacity to be of service and to contribute, is difficult for many persons to accept. It is a loss that many cognitively impaired persons simply do not accept. They continue to worry about paying the bills, feeding the children, and going to the office. Some find work and responsibility on their own, and even defend it from others who would take it over. We see a marked decline in the health and vigor of residents following the loss of a treasured role or responsibility. The activities program must recapture and preserve that experience.

The normal operation of a facility provides opportunities for residents to contribute: tidying, helping with food preparation, gardening, and distributing newspapers are a few examples. Most of these activities can be modified or broken down to suit the abilities of even very impaired persons, while still giving them the opportunity to be truly productive and to hear someone say, "Thanks." Small industries are another way to offer real work situations to persons with varying abilities. In one facility in Ontario residents prepare, bottle, and sell herbal vinegars. There is so much to do in the operation that a job can be found for everyone. Special projects offer individually suited opportunities, such as going out to do supervised volunteer work in the community (Arkin 1996).

There may be times when the only way to offer a work experience to very impaired persons is by contriving a simulated work project, such as folding towels that are never really used or pairing socks that the staff then unpair. Projects such as these should be used only with those residents who simply enjoy the process without concern for its actual application. Even then, special care must be taken that the "made-up" nature of the activity never becomes apparent to residents, and that their dignity in the face of visitors and other residents is diligently safeguarded. It is best to find activities that do not have this risk. Using the carpet sweeper is a bona fide chore with no risk of failure. Spraying the plants with a fine mister is another no-fail and useful chore. The mister and a cloth can also be used to freshen the handrails and doorknobs in the building. As the residential model of care is more and more accepted, contrived activity will become less and less of an issue, and program participants will have more of a real hand in the daily chores.

Self-Care

Personal care activities are the most private and intimate activities in our lives. We spend our early years mastering them, our middle years individualizing the way we do these things, and our later years just feeling comfortable about having things the way we like them. It is then, usually, that something happens to remove them from our control.

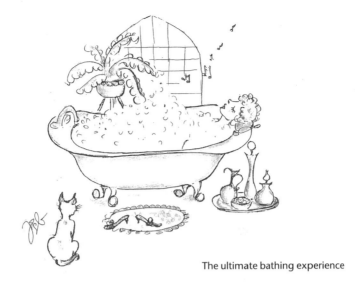

The ultimate bathing experience

Activities of daily living (ADLs) are the first activities over which we lose control when we come into a care situation. This is not really surprising, because the inability to perform these basic functions is the principal reason people come into care, and is the whole reason of existence for the medically based care facility. The assumption is that disabled persons need to have these things done for them and so it becomes the responsibility of the staff to dress, feed, bathe, groom, and toilet those who are in their care. It is their job, and they take ownership of these intimate activities. These precious intimate moments—for what can be more personal than choosing your own shade of lipstick, deciding when you've soaked long enough, deciding whether to shave, enjoying a good meal with friends, sitting over a bowl of cereal with the Sunday paper—become work. Even worse, they become someone else's work, and are often treated as a chore.

Because these precious personal activities fall under the jurisdiction of various departments (nursing, dietary, housekeeping), there is a concern that they be coordinated efficiently, to specified standards, and so they are set into a schedule, systematized, and depersonalized. This is a deep tragedy because, first, the person with Alzheimer's disease is reliant on caregivers to provide the best possible experience, and is usually unable to express preferences, offer alternatives, and compensate for losses. Second, ADLs are the most sensual, personally affirming, and socially stimulating activities available to a person on a regular basis. Third, ADLs

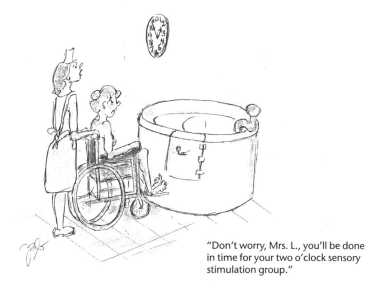

"Don't worry, Mrs. L., you'll be done in time for your two o'clock sensory stimulation group."

use old skills, so there is no need to teach new rules. The problem with this is that we must know what the old skills are. They are not often the same skills that are necessary for coping with the institutional way of doing things.

We know that there is a problem when people lose control over their own ADLs, because so many of our activity programs aim at trying to fill these needs. We set up socialization groups, sensory stimulation programs, grooming programs. It can lead to some pretty absurd situations.

Meals are often the highlight of a person's day. They should be treated as the important activities that they are. A meal, for a dependent person, represents valuable time in a one-to-one relationship. It can be a social experience if the meal is shared. It should always be a pleasant sensory experience.

Every meal offers an opportunity for programming activities. It can be used to build relationships among participants, to offer occasion for reminiscence, and to reinforce old, and perhaps neglected, social skills. A "breakfast group" can meet regularly. A program of regular family-style meals can be a "lunch bunch" or "dinner at our place." A wonderful thing happens when staff members participate, not as supervisors, servers, monitors, or feeders, but as people at the table enjoying a meal together. The sharing of a meal breaks down the "we-they" barrier between staff and residents and goes a long way to building the trusting, respectful relationships that pay such dividends in the long run.

Leisure

The dictionary defines *leisure* as "free time to enjoy one's ease, without pressure or demands." Although most activity rosters are made up mainly of leisure-type activities, the individual's time for leisure, in its true sense, must also be respected. For many persons this must also include time for quiet, contemplation, thinking, or just being. Sitting at the window and watching the birds is quite different from passively sitting in a group activity. By definition, the former is a meaningful activity, while the latter is not. Caregivers must be careful that, in their zeal for active programming, they do not take residents away from activities that are meaningful to them and force them into situations that have no meaning.

Activities Offered in the Environment

The Physical Environment

At the beginning of this chapter we mentioned that cognitively impaired persons need activities that come to them, engage them directly and spontaneously, and fit into their normal routine of life, not a schedule. This is exactly the kind of activity that a well-designed environment can offer. The physical environment stimulates some kind of activity, whether caregivers intend it or not. It can be restless pacing, fretting, calling out, removing and dismantling fixtures, hoarding, and rummag-

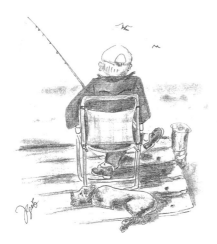

There is something to be said for simply enjoying the moment. Isn't that what leisure really is?

ing, or it can be exploring, strolling, visiting, observing, gathering, fixing, and sorting.

Walkways with stopping points and destinations encourage exploration, rest, and purposeful walking. Furniture groupings, especially of tables and chairs, encourage spontaneous socialization. Windows looking onto active areas such as streets, parking lots, or playgrounds attract and hold attention. Designers must be conscious of the fact that most people cannot see over the sill of conventionally situated windows. The only view many get from their chairs is of the sky.

Indoor work stations should include papers, magazines, and other interesting, safe, and replaceable objects to handle and explore. Because such items are likely to disappear or find their way into the permanent possession of residents, they should be considered consumables on the program budget. Large books and binders of mounted pictures tend not to stray so easily. A carpet sweeper can be left out for anyone who wants to tidy up.

A digging plot, clothesline, and potting shed are examples of outdoor features that can stimulate activity. One rural facility offered the gentlemen a tractor on which all the removable parts had been fastened. It was hoped that they would tinker with it. The gentlemen knew better what to do with an old tractor, though; they just went out and leaned on it while they gazed up at the sky and speculated about the weather.

The advantage of activities generated by the physical environment is that they happen spontaneously. There is no need to collect people, book a room, and set aside a period of time. It does, however, require persistent vigilance from every member of the staff and a commitment from each one to use these opportunities. The window may be there, but unless the caregiver who brings the wheelchair-bound person into the room positions her near it, there is no activity. This is really how the responsibility for activity programming should be shared.

The Social Environment

Every personal encounter is an opportunity for meaningful social activity. A word, a smile, "please," "thank you," "would you mind," or "please excuse me" can make a simple act such as removing a tray from in front of a person or passing a mop under his feet an opportunity for him to feel respected, loved, loving, in control, and a part of things.

A person who sits in the lobby to greet and be greeted by passersby is participating in a meaningful social activity that makes him feel valued, in control, and a part of things. Are these not, after all, the primary objectives of an activity program? What a pity when this wonderful pastime is misconstrued as a nuisance. Fire regulations prohibit wheelchairs near the exits. Administrators are uncomfortable when visitors are greeted by groups of residents who seem to have nothing to do but sit. So the residents are gathered up and brought down the hall to the activity room, where they have only one another to look at and where the activity staff try desperately to engage them. In the process a wonderful activity has just dissolved.

A valuable resource was created when the administration in one facility gave up an office near the lobby, took down the wall, and made an alcove with sofas, plants, and a fish tank where residents could sit and enjoy the passing parade with administrative sanction.

The Cultural Environment

Any group of people who live and work together develop a certain way of being, a commonly held set of values and traditions, essentially a culture. In an environment that accommodates vulnerable people, it is especially important that this culture be accepting, inclusive, and positive, and that it reflect equally the ethnic, spiritual, and cultural backgrounds of both residents and staff. The activities program is a powerful vehicle for molding and articulating this culture. It is a concrete expression of "who we are, what we do, and how we do it." The activities program can create and support allegiances through teams and even sports events. In Pittsburgh, the Adult Day Care programs formed a league of board hockey teams. Teams from various day programs visited one another and held tournaments. Membership, a sense of belonging, comes through participating in clubs and group projects. Chapter 12 describes how a group of very impaired residents developed a sense of membership. Traditions evolve through celebrations and recurrent events. A sense of identity and role comes from individual and group responsibilities in various activities. This is the process by which a community is built. It is such an important function that it must include everyone, even the most impaired, in a positive and affirming manner.

"Boxed" Individual and Group Activities

"Boxed" activities are tasks or pastimes that are known by everyone on the unit or in the program as being either comforting or interesting to a particular person or group of people. Such activities are available so that any staff member, family member, or visitor can take one out and offer it to the participant or do it with her. These activities are identified by gathering information from family about the person's past interests, spending time with the person, trying things and obtaining feedback, finding out how things work and documenting them, and then sharing them with other staff members at care conferences. The activities that are identified as working well with a person are then included in that person's care plan. They are usually simple things, like listening to a particular tape of music on headphones, looking at interesting picture books, doing puzzles, sorting various items, and playing cards. They can be work-related activities such as "paperwork," chores like digging compost into a garden, or reading catalogues. They can be specially assigned responsibilities. Although the activities staff usually take the initiative in identifying these activities and making the needed items available, once an activity is in place, it becomes the responsibility of anyone who is available at the appropriate time to bring it out.

Activities such as these can also be designed for the unit or program as a whole. One activity used very successfully by an activity coordinator in Canton, Ohio, was called the Walkers' Club. The coordinator would come onto the unit with a portable tape player and a tape of march music, pass out red vests (baseball caps would do), and take everyone who was inclined out for a walk. The vests identified members to each other and made it easier for them to stay together. They also identified members who might stray off to staff on other units so that they could direct them back to the group. The music was a familiar cue to start the activity, as it was always the same. It also kept the group together in spirit as well as in body. Once the activity became familiar to the residents, any staff member could take the walkers out.

When such activities are identified, tried out, and learned at a time when the staff are available and the participants are receptive, they become part of the unit lore. The residents or participants learn the rules comfortably. Because they are proven quantities that are known to work the staff are motivated to use them. They are also available as diversions when things are tense or when staff need to occupy several residents in order to deal with a crisis. If, for example, a person is feeling restless or is preoccupied with leaving, a staff member who knows that she enjoys a particular piece of music can easily offer her a set of headphones and a Walkman with her favorite tape already cued up. If several staff are needed to handle a situation, one staff member can easily start the march music, hand out the vests, call a meeting of the Walkers' Club, and take half the residents off the unit or out of the program.

Activities Programs

The activities that generally come to mind when we speak of activities programs are the planned, scheduled events that have always been the responsibility of the activities staff. Let us not be seduced into thinking that all good programs must be innovative and exciting or that everyone's being obviously busy means that the program is good. The only true measure of the program's effectiveness is the moment by moment satisfaction and pleasure of each participant.

There is a lot to be said for the old and the familiar, especially in the care of persons with Alzheimer's disease. There is as much value in quiet, subdued activities, such as a good sit in congenial company, as there is in an obviously social or physical activity.

Activities Must Be Planned on an Individual Basis

An activity program is planned not as an independent entity but on the basis of a stated philosophy and aim. The aim must be to meet the needs of, interest, and accommodate the abilities of each participant. That takes individual planning. Although there might be an overall plan, each individual's participation must be treated separately in terms of certain variables: the intent of the activity, what we would like to see the person gain from it, what strengths he will be able to exert in this activity, what disabilities must be accommodated, at what level he will participate, and which activities are appropriate for him. Otherwise we run programs and try to fill them. We write program goals that try to fit participants into the programs instead of the other way around. This approach can be frustrating to both the staff and participants.

The Intent of the Activity

The most important question we can ask ourselves about a program activity is "Why?" Why is this person here? If we do not know why we are doing something and why we are offering an activity, we have some thinking to do, because the purpose of the activity will determine how it is presented and how the resident is to be engaged. An example is a craft activity. It is close to Valentine's Day, so the schedule says that we will make Valentine's Day cards in the craft room. Everyone is welcome; a number of people are brought down without knowing what they will be doing. There is red cardboard, lace, hearts, flowers, scissors, glue, and sparkles. Some participants make nice cards. Others are helped to make nice cards. Some sit while staff make nice cards. Some get their fingers into the glue and sparkles and really do not know what is going on. Why are we doing this? Because it said so on the schedule.

If, however, we know that we are doing the activity because this is the time to express a loving sentiment to a person we hold dear, then the activity takes a completely different direction. We know that several residents can make beautiful cards, and we ask them to make a number of them for the event. Or we buy them. Several weeks or days in advance we ask families to bring pictures of people who are or were special to our participants. We spend the group time talking about these people, maybe thinking of notes to put into the cards. We help participants write these special thoughts into the cards that are either sent to the person, kept to give at a visit, or just tucked away as a special memory. The activity has meaning when we know why we are doing it.

Awareness of the intent of an activity also helps determine whether the activity will be done with a group and, if so, how large a group, or individually. Chapter 12 has more information on groups and group process.

Accommodate the Strengths, Deficits, and Needs of Each Participant

If this kind of programming is to be successful, it must address the needs, strengths, and liabilities of each participant. That requires ongoing assessment of the participants' abilities, and a deep and abiding respect for their retained abilities and life experience. Chapters 3 and 4 deal with the importance of personal history information and ongoing assessment.

Accommodating those abilities requires a process of individual planning once again. How will each person participate? One process of accommodating various levels of ability in one activity is called activity grading. This process assigns different roles to the participants, depending on their abilities and interests.

Another way to accommodate varying or declining abilities is to choose activities based on the level of their difficulty.

- Group activities are more demanding of attention than one-on-one activities.
- Activities in which only one correct response is possible are more demanding than those that allow for any response.

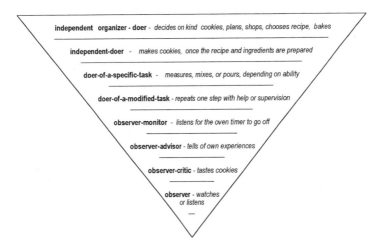

Activity grading makes it possible for many participants to enjoy an activity such as baking cookies despite varying levels of ability.

- Activities that demand active participation are more demanding than activities in which passive participation is possible.
- Activities that require sensory interpretation are more demanding than those which require only sensory appreciation.

For example, responding to quiz answers in a group is among the most demanding of activities, whereas listening to music with a friend is among the least. Therefore, as the person's condition progresses, activities would consist of those done in smaller groups, in which any response is as correct as any other, or which require no active participation and little sensory interpretation.

Guidelines for Choosing and Presenting Activities

Activities that are most often successful with cognitively impaired persons

- use old familiar patterns of movement;
- have a strong, rhythmic component;
- consist of one repetitive step;
- give immediate feedback;
- engage the person directly; and
- are fairly rigid, concrete, and predictable.

In presenting the activity,

- use the person's retained abilities;
- minimize distractions;
- limit options;
- avoid ambiguities;
- give step-by-step instructions and be consistent;
- give concrete visual cues; and
- eliminate the chance of failure.

To engage the reluctant person,

- don't ask but rather direct and inform;
- give strong, concrete cues;
- initiate the activity with the person watching;
- trigger an automatic reaction; and
- be sure that the activity is within the person's ability to understand and perform.

In coping with failure, you want to

- protect the cognitively impaired person from any further experience of failure;
- deflect or share the responsibility for the failure, but do so realistically; and
- measure success or failure only by the person's standards.

If the outcome is uncertain, prepare for possible failure so that the client cannot assume that it was his fault.

What Does It Take?

Several essential features or components underlie successful and effective programs. These are:

1. A commitment to a philosophy of programming whose aim is to enable each participant to continue doing those things and living the life that he would choose if he were still able.

2. A commitment to the concept of extraordinary respect and concern for the experience of each program participant. This means that the staff must be critical practitioners who feel supported in offering alternatives to practices that they feel are not respectful to either the residents or to themselves.

3. Cross-departmental flexibility and collaboration, a willingness to relinquish boundaries and fuzzy roles between nursing, activities, housekeeping and dietary.

4. Skill in ongoing assessment. This is not a matter of conducting one assessment and filing the results, nor is it finding out what a person can or cannot do. It is being constantly aware of how a person is responding to a situation in which he has been placed. It means knowing that person's abilities in terms of memory, language (receptive and expressive), attention, abstract thought, judgment, motor planning, and perception. An outline for ongoing assessment of these areas is included in Chapter 4. Ongoing assessment produces answers to questions such as:

    ■ Does the person have all the skills demanded of this situation?
    ■ Which does he have?
    ■ Which is he lacking?
    ■ How is he attempting to compensate for the deficit?

5. A system for information gathering. This is absolutely vital, because we are dealing with an area in which very strong old habits are already present. Unless we know what they are, we will be unable to use them and may even be going contrary to them. It can be as simple as using the right kind of makeup for each person if you are going to do a beauty group, knowing the standards of grooming that the person maintained, the preferred music or a special interest.

6. A forum for sharing information. Sometimes staff learn things during the course of an activity and need to share it so that others can implement it in their interactions and activity programs. Sharing includes

    ■ giving frontline staff access to notes, both recording and reading,
    ■ leaving notes on routines in strategic places,
    ■ placing personal articles in the person's room.

7. Skill in applying enabling techniques, environment, and equipment. These can be adaptations that staff make when they have been trained, or those learned from their own insights. Examples of enabling techniques are

    ■ giving step-by-step instructions,
    ■ warning,

- redirecting,
- cuing, and
- initiating.

An enabling environment offers

- appropriately orienting and familiar cues,
- reduced distractions, and
- privacy for both individuals and groups.

Enabling equipment may include

- furniture that enhances accessibility and seating posture,
- easily handled tools, and
- utensils for dining or tea programs.

When such supports are in place, all staff become members of the programming team. They all have the skills, commitment, and mandate to engage residents and participants in meaningful activity throughout the day, and in doing so they should also have fun together.

Most activities that are offered to persons in long-term care or day programs are done in groups. Those who cannot tolerate the large, often heterogeneous, group experience receive one-to-one attention. This way of thinking does not respond to individual needs. The compelling reason for setting up a group should be to offer the person who needs and desires it a meaningful social experience. Therefore, the group must be designed to meet the needs of the person, not the other way around. Unfortunately there has not been much attention given to group work with persons who have dementia. Perhaps this is because their needs are very special, and such groups require a lot of nurturing to produce results. Once it is done well, though, the outcome can be a wonderful lift for everyone involved.

Because dementia tends to isolate an individual, a positive social experience is particularly valuable. It offers membership, that is, being part of something, while still allowing individuals to maintain their unique identities. As a member of a group, a person acquires power and control, and is able to effect change and make an impact. In a group of peers, a person finds allies and mutual support. The group validates its members. They find solidarity and the thrill of consensus. The group also gives members feedback, expressing acceptance or rejection. The main reason why persons with dementia need special group programs is that the feedback they receive from mixed or ad hoc group experiences is all too often negative.

The Purpose of the Group

A number of people brought together to do a common activity is not a group. Unless the participants can somehow connect with each other, they are merely a number of people doing the same thing. Most real groups develop from a common interest. People come together to share information or to resolve a common problem. A person with dementia is at a disadvantage in a normal group because of limited ability to participate. Any stated purpose, be it discussing current events, reminiscence, arts and crafts, whatever, immediately imposes a standard of participation. It requires a form of compliance, and so inherently creates the possibility of failure.

The kind of group in which a person with Alzheimer's disease can thrive is one that permits the person to just be there and participate on whatever basis he is able. A group that permits this most effectively is one that exists simply to bring together a company of friends—in other words, a group with no agenda stated at the outset or imposed by the leader or facilitator. When there is no objective other than being there, everyone can participate. This may be a challenging concept for staff, who often feel compelled to operate with clearly stated, measurable, and action-oriented objectives.

Group Membership

Most activity group programs have an open membership. However, a group with an unpredictable membership is difficult for a cognitively impaired person. This person functions best in a closed group, with a selected and exclusive membership with which he can eventually become familiar and, hence, comfortable.

The most effective number for a group is six or seven. There might be some concern about justifying such small groups when the schedule of an activity coordinator must accommodate so many. But consider the following: A one-hour group program that involves thirty people may be done every day. It takes a good half hour to bring everyone together. With such a large number, the facilitator must give individual attention to keep members attentive because the setting does not promote initiative and interaction among participants. Each person may get two minutes of attention that has no context, usually catches the person off guard and has uncertain benefit. It may even be an unsettling and destructive experience; it certainly does not accomplish anything. This format is suitable for a fitness class, but not for a social group. On the other hand, a small group program offered to six compatible persons twice weekly for a half hour requires the same amount of staff time and offers each member a full hour each week of meaningful interaction. It also forms relationships, and builds confidence, identity, and belonging.

Who Leads?

Traditionally, a staff member is identified as the leader. This actually impedes the formation of a group, as all communication passes through the leader, and the participants usually leave all initiative to the leader. When the staff member's role is redefined to be that of facilitator, the group eventually takes on its own leadership. People speak up spontaneously. The topic of conversation is dictated by each person's initiative, by each one's interests and, therefore, remains consistent with each person's particular level of ability. Leadership can then shift from one member to another as the needs of the group and available resources dictate.

Initiating a Group

Most groups of dependent persons are started by someone bringing people into a room. This does not automatically make a group. Because of memory loss and impaired insight, participants may need to be told that they are there to be in the company of friends. This purpose usually needs to be restated frequently.

A group can also gather around a nondirected activity. I offered a nonstructured group program to several very impaired persons by bringing in a bag of interesting objects and simply putting it on the table. I then invited the designated members to come and see what I had brought that week.

Nurturing the Group

Each time the members come together, they need to be reintroduced to each other and to the group. Eventually the sense of membership evolves. The facilitator reinforces their ownership of the group at every opportunity, and validates each member's contribution and the achievement of the group as a whole. In this way, the facilitator focuses the group's development, and safeguards the process by mediating differences, compensating for disinhibitions, and enabling communication among members. The facilitator also acts as a model of social behavior that sets the tone of the gathering. Some of the most difficult yet rewarding things that the facilitator must do are to sit back, give the process time, let the members find their confidence, and watch the group grow.

Very impaired persons who are unable to interact need a facilitating medium. One of the most successful formats I have ever used is a "volley-ball team." A number of selected residents, most of them in Geri-chairs, are brought into a circle. The facilitator greets each one, suggests that they might try a game of volleyball, and starts off by tossing an inflated balloon to the person who is most likely to respond. With each toss, the person's name is said and every reaction, no matter how slight, is ac-knowledged. Each participant can react to or ignore the balloon, as he or she wishes or is able. No one is told what to do. No one's hand is ever moved forcibly to bat the balloon back. No one ever feels any pressure to do anything but what he wants to do. It is how people start to react on their own. They say things like, "I haven't done this in years." When the game is over, usually after about half an hour, the facilitator thanks people and tells them when the next practice is. When there is no pres-sure and only positive regard, people's abilities come out. Our fourth-floor volleyball team met regularly. Practices were posted on the activity schedule. The most fun for staff was seeing the reaction of off-floor staff and visitors when they were told who the volleyball team members were.

Outcome

Despite the fact that such a group starts off with no agenda or stated objective to accomplish and operates with little or no specific direction, eventually wonderful things happen. Participants learn, in time, that there is no failure here and, therefore, no risk in speaking up. They can try old skills and only positive feedback will result. So they speak up, share, reach out, and a group forms.

The facilitator also learns valuable lessons. One is the value of si-lence. Another is to trust that the participants, often with very limited skills and abilities, can bring something valuable to the situation if only they are given the time and the room to do so.

The Tea Group: A Special Program for "Difficult" Residents in Long-Term Care

Scott Peck (1987) prefaces his book *The Different Drum* with a story that he calls "The Rabbi's Gift":

A monastery had fallen upon hard times and only five old monks struggled for survival in their run-down mother house. In the woods close to the monastery was a hut in which a rabbi from the nearby village occasionally came to meditate. One day the abbot decided to seek counsel with the rabbi and set off into the woods. Unfortunately the rabbi had no advice for the abbot; and could only commiserate. Attendance at the synagogue in the village, he said, had also fallen off. As they parted, the rabbi said to the abbot, "The Messiah is among you."

The abbot returned to the monastery and told the monks of the rabbi's parting statement. As the monks puzzled over the cryptic phrase, they realized that each of them had some quality suggestive of the Messiah. So, just in case he was speaking to the Messiah, each of the old monks started to treat the others with extraordinary respect. By the same token, just in case each monk, himself, was the Messiah, they started to treat themselves with extraordinary respect as well.

The villagers who came to have picnics on the lovely grounds of the monastery occasionally went into the dilapidated chapel to pray and to meditate. Somehow, without being conscious of it, they sensed the extraordinary respect that radiated from the monks and seemed to permeate the atmosphere of the monastery. This wonderful feeling compelled them to bring their friends also. Soon, young men of the area started to come and ask to join the order. As knowledge of this place spread, more young men came; and, with time, it became once again a thriving order and a center of light and spirituality in the land.

The small group program described in the following pages draws on some of the principles of "community" that are presented by Dr. Peck and others. It was designed to help very impaired and difficult nursing home residents and the staff who care for them to find some common ground and establish a more positive living relationship.

Opzoomer et al. (1989) showed that 53 percent of nursing home residents have some degree of dementing illness. A study conducted at the Perley Hospital in Ottawa (Cowan 1989) revealed that 52 percent of cognitively impaired residents posed behavior-related problems. Experience indicates that a good many of these residents have behavior problems that are severe enough to exclude them from regular group activities within the facility and deny them the comfort of meaningful relationships with either staff or other residents.

These residents are described by a variety of labels. Feil (1982) referred to them as the "maloriented old old." Edelson and Lyons (1985) wrote about the "severely mentally impaired." Among staff and other residents, they are often referred to as the "biters, scratchers, screamers or kickers." Concern for these residents' needs is reflected in the literature about special group programs (Gilewski 1986). The programs described use a variety of modalities, including sensory stimulation, reality orientation, and even psychotherapy. Most of the programs described have produced positive results, but few endured without the support of a leader from outside the facility. Some were introduced as research projects, while others were special interest programs initiated by professional consultants from outside the facility. Unfortunately, when the researcher or consultant left, the program usually collapsed. Inadequate numbers of appropriately trained and committed in-house personnel and a negative or nihilistic attitude among staff have been cited as the main barriers to positive, sustained programming for very impaired and "behavior problem" residents (Burnside 1984). The absence of appropriate programming draws both residents and staff into a spiral that leads to more negative behavior and, eventually, staff burnout (Heine 1986).

The tea group program responds to two identified needs: the need for a program format to which very impaired, "behavior problem" residents can respond positively, and that nursing home staff can conduct without continued professional input; and the need for an in-house educational resource that helps staff develop a more positive and hopeful attitude toward these residents.

Program Rationale

Based on the traditional ritual of the tea party, this program puts residents into a familiar setting that naturally facilitates competent social behavior. The ritual of gathering to make, serve, and drink tea is almost universal. Its protocol provides the context and the cues that enable even very demented residents to perform in a remarkably competent manner.

Staff who participate in the program see these competencies emerge and learn that there is another side to these residents. They also learn how to promote these competencies in other areas of performance. The daily routine on the average nursing home floor offers both staff and residents few such opportunities; in fact, this routine usually does more to defeat the potential of these residents than to enhance it.

A Need Identified

The first tea group was started at the Medex Care Centre in Ottawa in 1987 and has continued to run despite three changes in facilitator. Most of the information described in this chapter is derived from that experience.

The Psychogeriatric Clinic at the Ottawa General Hospital had received a number of referrals for patients with very difficult behavior. They were all severely demented women whose cognitive impairment contributed to their hostile defensiveness or withdrawn behavior. Despite their cognitive impairment, each seemed to need an opportunity to share, to experience control, to reaffirm a positive identity and, most important, to have respite from failure and negative feedback. The staff who cared for these women were stressed and showed it in their approaches toward them. They needed an opportunity to encounter these women in a more positive context, to recognize in them the responsible, competent, and affable individuals that they once were. They also needed to learn how to facilitate the women's old competencies, but they needed to learn these skills under circumstances that did not threaten their own sense of competence on the job.

Program Design

The program was based on three premises: (1) these residents would respond positively to an environment in which they felt safe, respected, and successful; (2) the techniques that create such an environment could be described in specific terms and taught to staff who might have little previous experience in supportive or therapeutic programming; and (3) the staff would carry the approaches and attitudes that they witnessed in the program over into their daily interactions with these residents on the unit.

At the core of the program design was the group protocol, which specified the group membership, the physical environment, the ritual, and the respective roles of facilitator, members, guests, and nonparticipating staff on the unit.

The successful operation of the program depended on the understanding and support of all the nursing home staff. This occurred on several levels. Front line, supervisory, and administrative staff all received an in-service briefing about the program and were consulted for their input. Although only one member of the nursing staff at a time could receive intensive training and learn to facilitate the group, all other staff members were to participate in the program on a rotational basis as "guests." In this way everyone would eventually be involved and, it was hoped, committed to the success of the program.

The training of the staff to carry on the program and later to train other staff was fundamental to this undertaking. As the first facilitator and trainer, I modeled specific approaches toward residents in the group and discussed them with the trainee after each session. This gave the trainee a chance to see the residents' response to different approaches and then, as cofacilitator, to practice them. In addition to learning how to work with residents, the trainee also learned how to introduce and coach staff members who came to the group as "guests." Within six months, the first trainee felt confident enough to conduct the program independently and assumed the role of facilitator. A new trainee-cofacilitator was assigned and I withdrew.

The Protocol

Group Membership

Membership was limited to a selected group of residents in order to promote a consistent environment and foster group ownership and cohesion. This also ensured that the level on which the group operated remained consistent with the participants' limited abilities. If higher functioning residents had been permitted to join, they would likely have taken over the program and the target population would have been excluded once again.

The selection of members was based on an informal interview by the facilitator and the staff's descriptions of the prospective member's behavior and perceived needs. Members were chosen because they did not participate in any other social program within the facility, were frequently in conflict with the institutional environment due to some degree of cognitive impairment, and were trying to cope with their impairment in a maladaptive way. The extent of their real disability was difficult to determine because of their resistance to any kind of formal assessment and because of the effects of the phenomenon of "excess disability" described by Brody et al. (1971). Another criterion was that each member was capable of some socially appropriate response, even if it was only when approached in a friendly, undemanding manner. None of the members was suffering from an untreated psychiatric condition.

Program Content

During the five years that the program has been in existence, its content has remained consistent. The group meets for thirty minutes once weekly on the unit which houses the majority of the participants. The principal activity of the program is always the making, serving, and drinking of tea, with all its attendant ritual and rules of conduct. No other project is ever introduced during the session. The conversation and relationships just evolve around this simple activity, but how it is done determines whether the program achieves its objectives.

The Physical Environment

The meetings are held in a room that is free of intrusions and interruptions. The table is set with a tablecloth and flowers or a centerpiece. The tea service, including the pot, sugar bowl, and creamer, teaspoons, cups and saucers, napkins, a kettle to boil water, a container of tea bags, and a tray of assorted cookies or snacks are on a sideboard. These articles are all important because their familiarity has the power to provoke old patterns of behavior and social competency (Zgola and Coulter 1988). The seating at the table is determined according to participants' needs and their likelihood of interacting positively or negatively with one another.

The Ritual of the Group

Ritual is important. Regular, consistent, and predictable cues help the cognitively impaired participants' habituation to the program. Ritual also promotes group cohesion and fosters a sense of control in the participants.

The process begins with the words that staff use to invite participants to the session. They say, "The tea group is meeting in the quiet room. We would be very pleased if you'd join us." These words have been the most likely to produce a positive response. They also promote a sense of inclusion. Attendance is voluntary. Although they may be encouraged to come for a trial only, no one is ever forced to come. Members who choose not to attend are told that their presence will be missed and their regrets will be relayed to the group. To promote predictability and minimize wandering, members are always escorted into the room in the same order.

The meeting is opened with formal introductions if membership is relatively new, or greetings if members are familiar with each other. Everyone's name is mentioned several times as they are encouraged to greet one another. Absent members are also mentioned, and the contribution of each participant to the last meeting is acknowledged. Whatever conversation or comments members initiate take precedence and the facilitator takes cues from them.

Then comes the making of the tea. All decisions, even seemingly trivial ones, such as whether the water has boiled sufficiently, are reflected back to the group for consensus. These nursing home residents are so unused to having their opinion sought that even such trivia are, at first, taken seriously. By constantly reflecting back to the group the facilitator builds up their sense of control.

The facilitator delegates as much of the activity as possible and asks participants to look out for each other's needs. The facilitator's objectives are to identify possible roles, draw out competencies, and promote interaction among participants.

The conversation evolves if the facilitator is patient and observant and lets things happen. Since just being in a pleasant place away from the din of the floor is sometimes all a person may want, silence is also acceptable. Once participants are comfortable and feel free to risk, they venture more ideas and things emerge more freely. The facilitator must resist the temptation to set up themes or bring in set topics as one would do for a current events group or other structured activity. Such a structure inhibits members from ever expressing themselves about things that are really important to them.

If a participant wishes to leave early, she is encouraged to stay, but if she can tolerate no more she is invited to say her good-byes, is thanked for her participation, and then is permitted to leave, accompanied by staff if needed.

When the meeting has come to a natural end, usually in about thirty minutes, the facilitator thanks everyone individually for coming and acknowledges her contribution. Members participate in as much of the clearing away as possible. Those who were unable or unwilling to come are visited with a cookie and a small cup of tea, if possible, and are given a short recap of the meeting. This reaffirms their membership.

After the meeting, the facilitator, trainee-cofacilitator and staff guest have a recap discussion. They make brief notes about each member's participation that help them to keep track of changes and serve as reminders of issues that require follow-up. Such follow-up may include a need to collect or clarify historical information about some of the members, or to resolve situations about which members may have complained.

Roles

The Facilitator

The role of the facilitator is to create a positive experience for the participants by promoting their sense of control, safety, identity, and membership. This is done by encouraging, accepting, and praising members' participation; directing their participation by encouraging the reticent and checking the talkative; and following, listening to, and using the ideas of others.

The facilitator is often an interpreter and arbitrator for the group. This may involve making sense of the garbled or unintelligible comments of aphasic residents or using quick thinking, humor and diplomacy to deflect and defuse provocative or even belligerent comments resulting from a member's disinhibition or poor judgment.

Enabling independence while ensuring safety and freedom from failure or embarrassment is probably the greatest challenge that faces the facilitator in a group such as this. This requires a great amount of faith and trust, vigilance, and ingenuity. For example, instead of wiping a participant's chin, the facilitator would hand the resident a napkin with a telling gesture. Even very impaired residents usually respond appropriately to this familiar cue.

Precautions should be taken to avoid disasters. During one session we served chocolate cake; unfortunately, eating the moist, crumbly cake took so much of the residents' concentration that no social interaction occurred. Clothing was soiled and the table was a mess. The participants had been defeated and demeaned by a challenge that was beyond their abilities.

Guarding the individual's self-esteem also means minimizing potential failure by avoiding open-ended and factual questions, and by asking for opinions and advice instead of facts. Mistakes should not be corrected unless the person, herself, realizes the error and is seeking to correct it. A major contribution to the success of this program is the fact that participants are never exposed to negative feedback of any kind.

Most important, the facilitator is the model and sets the standards for behavior. Those standards are the impeccable good manners and deferential behavior that are appropriate for a formal tea party.

The Members

The real hosts of the program are the residents, and it is up to the facilitator to reflect that reality to other staff, families, and volunteers so that they understand this and do not behave as though the facilitator were putting on a tea party for the residents. Because of their cognitive impairment, members are unable to assume the role of hosts independently, but they take their cues from the facilitator. Consequently, every effort is made to treat them as competent, respectable, and independent adults. In a long-term care facility, where virtually everything is done for the resident, there is little opportunity to experience this kind of individuality. There is even less opportunity to do something for others and receive genuine thanks.

The Guests

The role of staff who are invited as guests is to observe and to learn. Therefore, they behave as guests, allowing themselves to be served by the participants. Guests are asked to set aside their nursing instincts and refrain from making any helping gestures, such as wiping chins or tucking in bibs. They must watch the facilitator's techniques and observe the resulting behavior in the participants. The prime directive is, "Behave toward the residents as you would toward a neighbor to whose home you had been invited for tea, and see what happens."

Other Staff

The success of the program also relies on the understanding and respect of other staff who are on the unit. They are asked to avoid interrupting or, if they must interrupt, to excuse themselves appropriately. Impeccable manners are the rule here as well.

Unit staff must also prevent other residents from interrupting and must explain to them why attendance is restricted. Most importantly, they must respect the program as an important, therapeutic activity that is more than "just a tea party." Along with respect for the program comes respect for the participants and what they are doing.

Outcomes

The transformation that occurred during the initial weeks of the program was nothing short of miraculous. Within eight weeks we saw the emergence of humor, compassion, initiative, and cohesion. One lady observed that the group did not have a president and moved that we elect one. We did. Another suggested that we close the meeting with the Lord's Prayer. We did that too, and the sound of the prayer and the vision of these "hard ones" holding hands with heads bowed was beyond words. One lady who ate every meal with her fingers and never seemed to mind the mess she created, fussed when a little tea spilled on her dress; and another who never seemed to notice, let alone care about, anyone, consoled her and suggested that she just soak it in cold water when she got home. These residents had all come into the program as self-centered, isolated, and unconcerned individuals. Through the program, they learned to care about themselves and others.

Most of our members had progressive conditions. Although they made wonderful gains at the start as they shed their excess disability, most did eventually deteriorate. They stayed with the group until they could no longer attend comfortably and then were replaced. Participation in the program had given them additional months and, in some cases, even an additional year or two to use skills and experience relationships that otherwise would have been neglected.

Although its membership changed, the group as an entity endured. The remaining members wished the ill a speedy recovery, expressed their sorrow over the loss of those who had died, and welcomed new members.

Carryover of changes in the residents' behavior onto the unit was less striking. Without the support of the program's enabling environment, residents did not practice their newly awakened social skills, but there was a somewhat heightened awareness that surfaced once in a while. Members occasionally exchanged greetings when they recognized each other. When the facilitator came onto the unit, several would ask if it was Wednesday already.

Most of the staff who attended as guests noticed positive changes. They reported that the residents' posture was less withdrawn in the group and remarked on the hidden skills of individual residents. Several reported that they had learned to facilitate those skills to promote the residents' cooperation in their daily care. They also encountered aspects of the residents' personalities that they could respect and enjoy.

Those staff members who had negative, rigid, and defensive attitudes about "problem" residents reported no benefit from the experience and were not invited back as guests. Our initial impulse had been to include them among the first guests in an effort to change their attitude. We later found that it was best to leave these few staff to adopt the new methods from the others by "osmosis."

While the tea group has continued as a resident program for five years, its use as a training program lasted for less than a year. Due to staffing pressures that resulted from an ever-increasing care load, the "guest" component of the program was curtailed only a few months after I withdrew as trainer and facilitator. Many staff who had participated found that their ability to work with the residents had improved. Unfortunately, not enough of the staff had been involved to effect a unitwide change of attitude and approach.

Discussion

The tea group was conceived to operate on two levels: as a resident program with therapeutic aims, and as a staff training program with educational aims. As a client program, it aims to provide the residents with a social experience that will promote a sense of identity by reinforcing the real self rather than the sick-role self. It aims also to establish a bond and a sense of belonging among a group of peers, to permit them to exercise control and ownership, and to provide them with a forum in which to ventilate and resolve troublesome feelings. These aims are achieved by the application of techniques and the expression of philosophy; the techniques used are consistent with the current state of knowledge about the needs of cognitively impaired persons. The ritualized protocol responds to the demented person's need for consistency and predictability (Mace and Rabins 1981). The use of familiar objects provokes old patterns of social behavior. The opened agenda is consistent with the outcome of studies by Åkerlund and Norberg (1986), who found that demented residents responded much more positively when given the opportunity to choose their own topics for group discussion.

In philosophy, the tea group strives to restore the members' experience of community and combat the sense of disconnectedness that so often accompanies a move into an institution. There is a growing body of literature about nature and importance of community. The work of Barkan (1981) and of Peck (1987) is particularly applicable here. Barkan described the importance of community among elderly persons in long-term care. Although Peck did not limit his discussion to institutional care or the aged, his view of community is also reflected in the structure of this program.

Barkan identified three essential characteristics of a community: (1) it permits each member to share in a collective; (2) it provides opportunity for personal growth and development; and (3) it offers members a chance to do for themselves and for others instead of abiding in the role of service recipients. The tea group is more likely to function as a community if its facilitator and supporting staff remain mindful of these three characteristics. The program must provide a place where everyone belongs, is acknowledged, and is missed when absent. Every member's contribution must be valued, yet no one must feel pressured to earn value. Each person must have a chance to grow as a result of the experience. Personal growth is not limited to the acquisition of new skills or insights, but often comes from a regained appreciation for old skills and accomplishments, as well as a renewed respect for old values and roles. The occasion to do for one's self and for others is a central element in the tea group experience.

Peck's criteria for community are inclusiveness, consensus, realism, self-awareness, and safety. These are also reflected in the philosophy by which the tea group operates. It is inclusive in that the only requirement for participation is need. Being neither democratic nor dictatorial in its decision making, the group operates on the basis of consensus. This characteristic is reflected in the role of the facilitator, who may guide the group to consensus but has no leadership role as such. The group is realistic and permits everyone freedom to state his or her mind or to alter the course or perception of the group. The group is also self-aware in that members become conscious of the group as an entity and see its maintenance as their prime reason for coming together. The members are encouraged to become increasingly thoughtful about the group and to actively nurture and evaluate it. Most important, the group is a safe place to be. There is never any danger of embarrassment, rejection, or failure. Unconditional acceptance and freedom to be one's self are its essential characteristics.

As a training program, the tea group aims to promote a philosophy of care among staff that reflects respect for each resident as a worthy individual, yet does not threaten the staff's own sense of competence in the job. It concretely demonstrates to staff the residents' retained capacities and clarifies their roles vis-à-vis the cognitively impaired resident. The program also gives staff an opportunity to try different interpersonal techniques in a safe and accepting environment.

The program format is responsive to the staff's needs as adult learners by placing responsibility for learning directly into their hands and letting them acquire techniques and knowledge at their own rate and to whatever degree they are able (Thomas 1985). The importance of staff attitudes in humanizing care of the elderly is referred to repeatedly in the literature. The fact that attitude can undermine even the most lavishly funded programs and can overcome the effects of the most modest setting is well known. The most frequently proposed solutions are modeling and education. This group program supports the concept of changing attitude by modeling.

Although there have been few long-term changes in the residents' behavior on the unit as a result of this program, the group continues and noticeable changes have occurred in the residents while they are actively involved. There have also been subtle changes in the behavior of the staff who attended the program. Perhaps the most marked have been their appreciation for the residents' lifetime experiences and their awareness of the tremendous effect that environment and approach can have on a mentally impaired individual's abilities.

It is unfortunate that the structured training component of the program was sacrificed because of perceived workload pressure. In fact, it is perhaps one of the most effective and economical staff education and support options available. It would be wonderful if the positive and enabling atmosphere of the tea group were to permeate the facility, just as the extraordinary mutual respect of the old monks eventually permeated that troubled community.

13

When Is Breakfast?
Any Time You Want It

Deborah A. Macdonald Connolly, R.N., B.N.,
and Jitka M. Zgola, O.T.(C)

Meadowview is a special care unit at the Beechgrove Nursing Home, in Charlottetown, Prince Edward Island. It is home to forty-four residents. The majority of these residents have moderate to severe cognitive impairment. The unit operates with a stated philosophy. Three essential elements of that philosophy are:

- Despite their impairment, residents are to be treated as adults with unique life experiences.
- Each resident should be supported in the performance of activities of daily living to enable a maximum level of personal achievement.
- A calm, slow-paced environment that is people-oriented rather than task-oriented is the best support for that achievement.

Wouldn't It Be Nice?

In the fall of 1988 the staff of Meadowview had been meeting to review and discuss their philosophy. Although they felt positively about the philosophy itself, they were frustrated with their efforts to implement it. At about the same time, we were conducting a three-day seminar on dementia care at Meadowview. During one of the discussions, a simple yet provocative question was asked which brought into focus one of the sources of their frustration. We had been discussing old age and some of the freedoms one looks forward to as part of retirement, and the staff concluded that one such freedom was the opportunity to get up and have breakfast whenever you want it. The question that arose from that discussion was, "Wouldn't it be nice if residents could be given the same freedom?" By the time the seminar broke for coffee, the Meadowview staff had gathered and were expressing a wish to change the breakfast routine on the unit.

Deborah A. Macdonald Connolly was unit director on the Meadowview Unit at Beechgrove Nursing Home when this program was established.

How Things Used to Be

The established routine ran counter to each of the three basic elements of the unit's philosophy. It failed to acknowledge the individual habits, routines, and preferences that each resident on the unit had developed over a lifetime. With a rigid schedule that required them to report from 7:00 to 7:15 A.M. and serve breakfast in the main dining room or from the unit tray carrier at 8:15 A.M., staff were rushing frantically to wake, wash, and dress residents. As a result, staff had little or no opportunity to encourage that independence and personal achievement which was believed to be so important to residents. Finally, the routine evoked a task-oriented approach, not a people-oriented one. It created an agitated and often contentious atmosphere. Staff resented having to wake people to ensure that they would get their breakfast before the trays were returned to the kitchen. Residents often responded negatively to being rushed. A day that started in a rushed manner often led to a morning of restless, agitated behavior. A change was needed.

Planning a Change

The plan to change received momentum from having been staff-generated right from the start. At the very beginning, too, it was acknowledged that interdepartmental planning would be essential. With these convictions, a pilot program was set up.

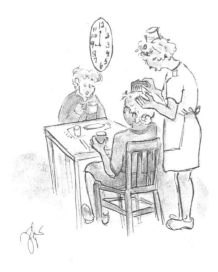

"Let's get your hair combed quickly
so you don't miss Beauty Group"

The program had to address a variety of habits and needs among the residents of Meadowview. A few residents were early risers who would wander about, hungry and restless, and were usually encouraged by staff to return to bed. Other residents who had been awake intermittently throughout the night or had fallen asleep only in the early morning hours were difficult to rouse at 7:30 A.M. Every resident had a certain capacity for contributing to his or her self-care if given the time and appropriate assistance. With these factors in mind, the following schedule was designed:

6:30 A.M.
Dietary staff bring coffee, muffins or biscuits, and fruit to the unit.

7:30 A.M.
Dietary staff bring carriers with bulk porridge (two kinds), eggs (plus special-order eggs), bacon, and six orders of toast.

9:45–10:00 A.M.
Dietary staff return carriers to kitchen.

10:00–10:30 A.M.
Continental breakfast again available.

The care routine that went along with this schedule ran as follows. Each staff member at Meadowview is responsible for the care of six to nine residents. Priority was given to ill or dying residents, who were checked first and their needs attended to. Staff would then go to the room of a resident from their assigned group who was already awake. They would help the resident to wash and dress. If the resident preferred to dress after breakfast, this option was also available, and he could go to the dinette for a continental breakfast if the main meal was not available yet. As other residents awoke, they would be assisted in washing and dressing and then were brought or came to the dinette and given breakfast in whatever manner suited their functional ability. For example, one resident might be given juice and porridge, while another could cope with only one item at a time. If no one was awake in a particular staff member's group, that staff member would go and help someone from another group.

Supports to Implementing the Pilot Project

The implementation of such a program requires a great deal of good will and cooperation among the departments involved, nursing and dietary. Several meetings were held with dietary and nursing staff. There was in-service training for those members of the dietary staff who had had little contact with the cognitively impaired residents. This was done to ensure that the staff were aware of the specific needs of these residents and how this program was intended to serve those needs.

In the week before the implementation of the pilot, a specially designated member of the dietary staff was assigned to work through the process from the dietary department's side, assigning specific duties and setting schedules. This person was chosen on the basis of her understanding of special care residents and her positive disposition toward the program. This same staff member remained on the unit for breakfast during the first week of the pilot to monitor and assist with the program. She also attended the daily meetings that were set up to evaluate it. She then withdrew in the second week of the program. During the third week, she remained available to dietary staff to wrap up any loose ends and ensure that they were secure with the program.

Immediate Changes

The sights and sounds of Meadowview in the morning underwent an immediate transformation.

6:30 A.M.

Before One or two hungry residents, up and ready to start their day, would be pacing the unit.

After These same residents are sitting in the dinette with a newspaper, enjoying juice or coffee and a muffin.

7:20 A.M.

Before Rushed staff, already feeling harried, ready to start the rush.

After Following report, relaxed staff check to see which residents are awake.

8:00 A.M.

Before Staff were still rushing, many residents impatiently waiting in the dinette for breakfast, some banging on the tables, others dozing, while still others were swearing at those who were making the noise. Other residents were being rushed to the main dining room or dozing in their chairs, waiting to be taken. Some of the residents who had been taken to the dining room early were now returning, some several times, without having had breakfast.

After   Very little noise! Some residents enjoying breakfast in the dinette, while others are still in bed or just getting up.

10:00 A.M.

Before   Staff were struggling to "finish" their tasks by coffee break, feeling frazzled. Residents were sitting with nothing to do, many of them restless.

After   Most beds are not made. No one is very concerned. Some residents are making their beds or puttering in their rooms, while others are still eating or dressing. Staff know that they can take the time they need and go for a coffee break when the residents' needs have been seen to. Many stay on the unit and have coffee with the residents.

Some Concerns: The Evolution of a Program

Following the six-week pilot, the program was deemed a success, and it was agreed to implement it on a permanent basis if it continued to work well over the next six weeks. As in any dynamic process, however, procedures continued to be refined and the program continued to evolve.

There had been concern that some residents might miss part of their breakfast in the less structured situation. In response to this concern, each staff member who had detailed knowledge of the preferences, needs, and habits of certain residents made up a list on each one. Each time an item on the list was served and eaten, it was checked off. A similar "procedure list" was posted in the room of each resident to assist staff who might be unfamiliar with a resident's morning care routine; this enabled all staff to provide the kind of assistance and support that would encourage an optimum level of achievement from the resident.

The potential for skin irritation among late risers with incontinence, especially in the warm summer months, had been a frequently raised concern when the program was first proposed. In fact, this never proved to be a problem; incontinent residents were checked during the night as usual, and this continued to prevent prolonged skin exposure to urine.

The question whether residents would continue to receive a balanced diet was also raised. Would the person who had a continental breakfast at 6:30 A.M. not be hungry before lunch? And would a breakfast eaten at 10:30 A.M. not interfere with lunch? In fact, most residents who ate the early breakfast were ready for another full breakfast at 8:00 A.M.; and those who ate late had only a light meal. A "night lunch" is served on the unit between 7:00 and 8:00 P.M. This is considered by some residents to be another meal. All told, the staff felt that there had been no change in the residents' intake.

How would nursing supervisors handle the distribution of medications if all residents were not up at 8:00 A.M. to receive them? The supervisors each worked out the best system for recording the residents who had not received their medications on the first pass, and would return later. Even before the program was instituted, it had not been uncommon for the nurse to return several times to a recalcitrant resident.

There was concern that imposing the tasks normally done by dietary staff would unduly burden nursing staff. In fact, nursing staff spontaneously started to take on additional dietary tasks, such as making fresh coffee and toast on the unit instead of waiting for it to come ready-made from the kitchen. Although they acknowledged that they were taking on more tasks, nursing staff all felt that they had more time than before the change.

Outcome

The Meadowview breakfast program has been in operation for two years. Staff were canvassed about how they feel about the changes in the morning routine. In retrospect, they all feel that mornings were rushed and harried. They recall their frustration and sadness at having to roust residents who they knew had not had a full night's sleep. The priorities identified by staff were to have people up and dressed. There was no opportunity to express regard for the individual's needs and wishes or to let residents do as much of their own care as they were able to. Although the morning care got done, the staff felt dissatisfied with the quality of the resident's experience and their own as well.

The reaction of residents to the original routine suggested that they too were frustrated and resentful. It was demonstrated in agitation, disorientation, persistent restlessness, and impatience.

With the program in place, staff noticed a more relaxed atmosphere on the unit, and felt relieved of the need to rush. They identified one of the main benefits as being the opportunity to give residents choices:

when they would get up, how much of their own care they would do and when they would do it, what they would eat for breakfast and when that would be. They also had the time to support the residents in carrying out these choices. More one-on-one time was spent with those residents who needed it.

Residents responded to the program by looking more relaxed. There was less resistive, combative, and difficult behavior. There was also a greater expression of individuality. Different people were doing different things at different times. Someone might be in the corner of the dinette, sitting with a friend and a cup of coffee. Someone else might be sitting by himself with his porridge and the paper, because that is the way he is accustomed to eating breakfast. Residents who can cope with only one item at a time might have just their juice, while others are able to manage a full setting.

There have also been other, more subtle, changes in the morning atmosphere. You seldom see a tray and never on a table. Trays are sent only to those residents who, for some reason, are having breakfast in their rooms. The noise level on the unit has dropped considerably. The smells on the unit have changed as well. It smells more like home. The smells of fresh coffee and sometimes even burnt toast have replaced the more usual combination of sleep, soiled bed linens, and toiletries.

Family members have expressed pleasure in the knowledge that their loved ones are being offered a choice which they themselves value in their own lives.

The program has also affected the way that staff see their responsibilities vis-à-vis the residents. It has reinforced their role as helpers in the residents' home and given credence to the philosophy that residents are to be treated with the respect accorded to adults and, therefore, be given as much autonomy as possible. The old routines created a conflict with this philosophy. Staff believed in one set of values, yet felt compelled to comply with another. The new breakfast program has permitted them to work according to their philosophy, and reinforced it by demonstrating a positive outcome.

Staff have also gained an enhanced appreciation for the simple, everyday activities in the lives of their residents. As part of the in-service training that accompanied the development of this program, staff were invited to participate in a short exercise (Zgola 1990). On separate pieces of paper, they were asked to make two lists: one of exciting, recreational activities (skiing, bowling, bingo, arts and crafts, etc.); the other, of more mundane tasks (dressing and grooming, caring for home and belongings, preparing a snack and sharing it with a friend, looking through the paper, puttering, pondering). Then they were to imagine themselves walking down the street with both lists in their pockets when, suddenly, the Grim Reaper appeared. "My friends," he would say. "Your time is up. But I will give you twenty more years if you give me one of those lists. Consider it carefully, though," he would caution. "You will never again be able to do the things on the list that you give me." The staff were asked which of the lists they would give up.

It was not an easy decision, but it demonstrated the relative value and, therefore, importance of daily living activities in anyone's lifestyle, including that of cognitively impaired residents. These are the activities that make a major contribution to an individual's sense of self and sense of control and purpose. Before the breakfast program residents were dressed, washed, and fed by 8:30 A.M., then spent the rest of the morning in a state of restless agitation or wandering about collecting other residents' belongings, while a harried staff member made their beds and tidied their rooms. There was a concern that a special activity program should be planned to give them something to do, something that would relieve the agitation and restlessness.

With the restructured morning, many residents are now able to rise at their preferred hour, have a continental breakfast in their housecoats or dressing gowns, or get themselves dressed and washed with help, if they prefer, before breakfast. With a calm, relaxed routine that is responsive to their need for autonomy, most are happy to putter about, making their beds, tidying rooms, or looking at the world go by until lunchtime. In fact, their routine is not very dissimilar to that of many senior citizens in the community, and there is no need for special activity programming. The breakfast program is the most natural activity there could be. This approach challenges some of our basic notions about long-term care, but we already know that the care requirements of persons with dementia in themselves pose a significant challenge to these notions.

Costs

Only two expenditures were associated with this program. Despite the increase in nursing staff's workload, there were no changes in the staffing pattern on the unit. During the week before the start of the pilot and for two weeks into the pilot, one part-time dietary staff member was assigned, at a cost of about $800. The equipment, two thermal containers from which the breakfast was served, cost $800. The thermal containers were chosen in preference to a steam table because of safety. Because it has no heat source of its own, the cart on which the containers were placed could be left unattended with no danger of unwary residents burning themselves. In addition, these containers could also be used for outdoor events to keep foods warm.

Another "cost" of the program was incurred in terms of staff losses. One staff member found she could not work comfortably with the lack of structure and asked to be transferred. Her request was honored. It must be acknowledged that this kind of work does not suit everyone. It is important that staff feel they have the freedom to express their feelings and ask to be allowed to use their skills and talents elsewhere.

Tips for Success

For such a change to come about successfully, it must stem from a conviction among the staff that it will enhance both their job satisfaction and the quality of life for the residents. Staff must be convinced of the impact that the environment, both human and nonhuman, has on cognitively impaired persons. They must also see how a change will fit into a philosophy with which they are familiar and which they support. Then the change becomes a natural step in the development of the program. There must also be cohesion and a feeling of team membership among the staff. A new program will not work unless it is perceived by a majority of the staff as a team effort.

Interdepartmental collaboration is another essential ingredient. Meetings and in-service training for dietary staff ensured positive support for the program. The dietary department also provided the extra staffing to get the program under way. The continuity provided by a staff member who was familiar with the eating habits and preferences of the residents was very important, since nursing staff seldom accompany the residents to the dining room. Having the same person available was also important at the beginning, because nursing staff rotate through shifts. Her presence helped to prevent frustration and insecure feelings on the part of the staff.

Families are also an important part of the team. They must be informed of any programming changes that are planned and receive a clear explanation of the intended benefits of the change. Otherwise, their reactions can place the whole project in jeopardy. Imagine the reaction of family members who come in and, without any explanation, see their loved ones not dressed, puttering in their rooms, sitting in their housecoats and looking at the paper with staff who are drinking coffee on the unit at 10 o'clock in the morning. When they were informed and could put the above situation into context, they were able to appreciate the thought, effort, and motivation that had gone into the program and supported it enthusiastically.

Evaluation meetings were held every day for a while. These provided staff with an opportunity to share feelings about the program, and to talk over the good things that had happened and those that would require change. Staff needed to know that they had a say and that their suggestions would be taken seriously. Only in this way would they acquire a sense of ownership of and a commitment to the program. There would be less temptation to say, "I told you it wouldn't work."

Conclusion

This program is presented as a model to illustrate creative, innovative, and challenging ways of providing residents in long-term care with an opportunity to experience some of the simple, mundane, yet vital aspects of daily living that are all too often taken for granted, but are vital to any meaningful existence. It is also presented to advance the concept that the needs of residents can and must take priority over the routines that were established to serve the needs of the institutions that house them.

14

I Have Him Dressed—What Now? Organizing a Day at Home with a Cognitively Impaired Person

Why Is Planning Necessary?

Time and energy are our most valuable assets. Whether they are well spent depends largely on what we do, how we plan our days and weeks, and where we set our priorities. Usually we do not look closely at why we do the simple, ordinary, day-to-day things in life. We seldom pay attention to setting them up to be really satisfying. Normally, we just go ahead and do the laundry, take a walk, garden, or take out the garbage. We save our planning for big things such as major projects, holidays, and celebrations. Alzheimer's disease puts a different spin on things. It interferes with a person's ability to remember, organize, start and stop appropriately, and complete even the simplest everyday task. Doing or not doing can become a major preoccupation of both the caregiver and the person being cared for. More than one caregiver has been brought to tears of exhaustion from trying to contain or redirect the restless activity of a person who just cannot settle to do anything but is perpetually on the go. By the same token, many have been demoralized by seeing a once active, dynamic person languish in inactivity. When we see this person gradually slipping into lassitude or pursuing seemingly aimless activity, we feel compelled to do something. We wonder if she is losing her interest and sharpness because of inactivity or lack of purpose. Would she regain that spark if we just encouraged her to take up old interests? Or is the inactivity and lack of direction a consequence of lost ability? If that is the case, then how do we compensate for disability so she can once again be active and productive?

It is very tempting to encourage the person who seems to be languishing in inactivity to just do more, try harder, take an interest. Talk and pushing the person achieve little, however. Knowledge, insight, and planning are a caregiver's best tools. In the interest of serving the needs of the caregiver as well as those of the person being cared for, it is worth

looking at what we do, why we do it, and how we can get the most
satisfaction from doing it.

The Value of Doing, and the Consequences of Not Doing

We instinctively know how important a normal level of satisfying
activity is to anyone. During any period of prolonged inactivity, such as
hospitalization, we experience disorientation and start feeling out of
touch. We tend to feel useless and without purpose. We also miss the fun
and pleasurable sensations that come from activity. We particularly miss
the satisfaction of a job well done, that precious sense of accomplishment and success. These are the things that we would like to recapture
for the person in our care. Seen in this light, activity is more than an
escape from boredom; it is a major aspect of living. Activity keeps a
person tuned in to the world around her. The routine of the day's activity
orients her to time and place. Activity keeps a person in touch with
others and provides much needed sensory stimulation. Doing something, being useful or helpful reinforces a person's sense of personal
worth. There are also many activities that just feel good, and that we do
just for the fun of doing them.

We can get some idea of what losing the capacity to do is like by
walking, for a moment, in the shoes of a person who can no longer do.
Imagine that you still have the energy and the desire to do things, but
have lost the ability to organize, plan, initiate, and successfully complete
even the simple tasks of daily living. You don't know what is wrong, but
sometimes, when people ask you to do something, you are not sure
exactly what they want. Sometimes it is just impossible to get a task
started. Other times, when you try to do something, you get into a mud-
dle. You get involved, anticipating a sense of accomplishment or just
enjoying the pleasure of doing, but things go wrong. People think that
you are being negative, uncooperative, or even spiteful. This leaves you
isolated, with nothing that you can do confidently, no way to express
your talents and abilities, affecting nothing, useless and needed by no
one. You have no way to establish and maintain your social roles or just
to experience the satisfaction of a job well done. The result is often
withdrawal, frustration, restlessness, and many of the other behaviors
that are seen as part of Alzheimer's disease. By facilitating successful and
meaningful activity, we can help the affected person regain a sense of
identity, control, and efficacy. We can even, at times, actually improve

function by reversing the effects of a phenomenon known as "excess disability."

Breaking the Spiral of Excess Disability

Although we cannot reverse the course of Alzheimer's disease, we can undo and prevent the effects of excess disability. This term refers to a loss of function that exceeds the actual effects of the physical damage caused by the illness. It develops in the following way. Because a person's initial disability makes it difficult for her to interact effectively with a conventional environment, her behavior becomes anomalous and efforts to do things are often unsuccessful. Repeated failure and frustration eventually cause her to stop doing things and interacting with people. This leads to social isolation and sensory deprivation, which in turn results in more anomalous behavior, more deterioration in function, and even greater social and sensory deprivation. So it goes in an ever-downward spiral, until the person's functional decline far exceeds the effects of the original disability. When a person is supported in an environment that accommodates her disability and enables continued participation, we see the effects of "excess disability" peel away and function improve. This effect is described in "The Tea Group," a delightful experience recounted in Chapter 12. To provide such an environment, we must understand the factors that prevent the person from being able to do: in other words, the nature of her disability and the barriers that need to be overcome.

Some of the Reasons People Stop Doing, and How We Can Help

A practical insight into some of the obstacles that keep a person from participating or succeeding is essential if we are going to accommodate her in meaningful activities. The most common impediments are loss of initiative, inability to plan and execute complex tasks, failure to understand and make accurate sense of sensory stimuli, inability to focus attention and withstand distractions, memory loss, and loss of motivation. Following is a brief look at each of these factors.

Alzheimer's disease impairs a person's ability to think in abstract terms and, hence, to appreciate the need for action or determine the kind of action that is appropriate to the circumstances. It also impairs a person's ability to initiate an activity once she recognizes its value. The ability to get things moving is just not there. Under these circumstances she needs a physical boost to get started. Concrete cues, examples, and demonstrations of the activity will help. For example, she may say that she is hungry and wants to eat, but just sits in front of her plate. She starts to eat only when you have handed her the fork. The physical cue was what she needed to get her going.

Most activities require decisions at certain points. This requirement demands the ability to plan and execute a complex task, step by step, through its various stages. If the person who has difficulty in this area becomes hung up at a decision point and is unable to figure out what to do next, she may abandon the activity or go off in the wrong direction and encounter problems and failure. This is frustrating and can even lead to a catastrophic reaction. To minimize the chances of this happening, we can offer activities that have few decision points. Activities such as folding newsletters or stuffing envelopes are repetitive tasks comprising one or two steps with which the person can quickly become familiar and which they can do comfortably. Another alternative is to encourage tasks at which the person is already so skilled that decisions are no longer an issue, and the person moves automatically from one step to another. These are usually activities that the person has done for so long and so frequently that they have become "hardwired." A person who is very impaired otherwise may still be able to play piano, iron, or play a familiar card or board game.

Perceptual problems constitute another impediment. The person may not be interpreting what she hears or sees correctly, and that might not be obvious to others. Most people in the earlier stages of Alzheimer's disease retain good social skills and can give the appearance of understanding when in fact they do not. They can acknowledge that something needs to be done and even politely agree to do it. Later, when they fail to follow through, their caregivers wonder why. Another indication of possible perceptual disturbance is the person's inability to accurately identify objects necessary for a task, even when those objects are out and available. They may not be obviously positioned or in a clear line of sight, so that the person is unable to make them out. To circumvent problems of perception, we can double check that the person understands by asking for feedback occasionally, and we can make all stimuli clear and unambiguous.

The ability to focus attention, to withstand distraction, and to shift attention appropriately is essential to the successful participation in any activity. A person with deficits in this area will need an environment that is as free from distractions as possible. A caregiver must anticipate that the person is likely to wander away from a task if left unsupervised. The person is also likely to respond to environmental stimuli in a very concrete and direct fashion. For example:

> Mrs. X is dusting and doing quite nicely. As she finishes the dining room, she passes through the kitchen to go to the living room. On the way she goes by the sink, and in direct response to seeing the faucet, she turns it on, rinses out the dust rag that she has in her hand, and hangs it on the hook under the sink. That done, she loses track of the dusting, doesn't know what to do next, and goes off in search of her husband, who thought he had a few minutes to read the paper while she was busy. He asks her where the dust rag is. She has no idea.

Memory loss also makes it difficult for a person to stay on track with a task. Not remembering which steps of a task have been completed, she cannot anticipate what needs to be done next. A person with memory loss also finds it difficult to acquire new learning, or to adjust to changes and unfamiliar settings. This is one of the reasons why routine and a consistent environment are such a help to a person with Alzheimer's disease.

Loss of motivation, or inertia, can be quite striking in some cases, especially in persons who also exhibit a flat effect, that is, a loss of emotional expression. A person with diminished motivation is often content to just sit quietly on the periphery of activities. When she is asked if she wants to participate, her answer is usually a bland refusal with no ire or distress. When an activity is presented, she may participate as long as she is actively encouraged. Caregivers may consider it a failure when they are unable to keep such a person motivated, but as long as the person is experiencing no distress and not actively excluded or neglected, letting her participate passively is not unkind. In fact, continued prodding and encouragement to participate when the motivation is not there, may actually cause her more discomfort.

Whenever motivation lapses, one is inclined to wonder if the person is depressed. Depression and dementia are not mutually exclusive. Therefore, if there is any reason to suspect that a person is depressed, especially when loss of motivation is associated with sadness and/or irritability, this should be brought to the attention of the person's physician. The physician will either rule out depression or treat it appropriately. There are some general guidelines for distinguishing inertia from depression. A depressed person usually has a sad demeanor, may be irritable when asked to participate, will not bother trying to answer questions, and will just tell people to go away. A person with inertia and no depression is usually placid, likely to acknowledge that activities are a good idea, may even agree to do them some time, but takes no initiative. This person usually tries to answer questions, but may not have the correct information and generally does not express distress.

A Process for Thinking Things Through

Plan with an Eye on Your Own Needs

Far too many family caregivers become exhausted trying to keep their loved one active and involved, so much so that they have no time for their own lives. If a caregiver is to do a good job, she must see to her own needs too. One of those needs is time. Therefore, as a caregiver you should plan the cognitively impaired person's activities with an eye to having some time for yourself as well. Distinguish between activities that will occupy the person independently and that will give you a break, and those that you will do together. Unless you are clear about the difference and purposefully set things up that way, the activity will be a source of perpetual frustration. If you really need the time to yourself and find yourself repeatedly drawn into the activity to help or supervise, you won't get your needs met. Furthermore, the person you are caring for is likely to sense your irritation, disappointment, or impatience, and will become upset or apprehensive. The situation will be tense and dissatisfying for both of you.

Whenever you are going to do a task together, be prepared to give it your undivided attention. If you feel that the job is going to require your full attention, or that leaving the person in midcourse would likely lead to disaster, turn on the answering machine or let the telephone ring. It's a matter of priorities; put everything else aside and give yourself permission to spend an uninterrupted period of time doing just that one thing.

Make sure that the activity is something that you too can enjoy. One thing that caregivers must learn very early is that the only reliable source of gratification in the task of caring is their own satisfaction in doing it. There is no relying on the gratitude or appreciation of the person for whom you are caring. Although her appreciation is wonderful when it comes, it may be expressed very seldom, if ever. It cannot be the sole source of a caregiver's motivation. You have to do this simply because it is something you want to do. So, give yourself the edge by choosing activities and tasks to do together that are a pleasure for you too.

What Can the Person Derive from the Activity?

We usually think that the main reason for doing anything is to have it done. The things that we do for pleasure tend to be the extras, the frills, the reward. In dementia care this can no longer be our reasoning, because things are not likely to get done the way we think they should be, and because without memory, the ability to anticipate satisfaction (i.e., deferred gratification) no longer exists. If there is any pleasure to be gained from an activity, it must be from the doing, not from the having done. There is no such thing as present pain for future gain. Therefore, the primary reason for participating in an activity is to experience the pleasure of doing it.

This is not to say that everything must be jolly fun. One of the most overlooked pleasures in doing, and one of which the dependent person is most deprived, is the pleasure of being helpful and productive. We hear the words "could you please" and "thanks" so often that we come to take them for granted. It usually means that someone wants us to do something for them, and we might even find it to be an annoyance. But imagine how wonderful these words must sound to a dependent person who is always on the receiving end of a relationship, and who may now feel helpless and useless. These are the benefits of activity that we want to make available to an impaired person. They are simple pleasures but invaluable ones. They are easy to overlook when we experience them regularly, but devastating when they are missing from our lives.

Value the Little Things

What kinds of activities can fill these needs for a person whose abilities may be very limited? They need not be special or exciting things. Usually, if given their due, the simple everyday experiences of living are the most fulfilling. Think of a day when you feel that you've done nothing of consequence. What have you really done? Got up, dressed yourself, chosen your color of lipstick or shaved, had a cup of coffee, looked at the paper, greeted a neighbor, looked at the garden, shoveled some snow, washed the dishes, folded some laundry, taken a walk. These are simple things that can bring pleasure, orientation, sense of purpose, identity, and control to a person. Sitting and looking at the sunset, sorting through a drawer of old stuff, or watching the birds at a feeder are

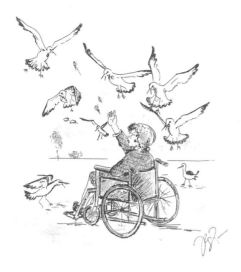

Mrs. Jordan's dining group

activities that need little in the way of attention, memory, or organizational ability, yet can bring a lot of satisfaction.

Recognize Various Levels of Participation

Even complex tasks can offer a disabled person an opportunity to participate if we consider different levels of participation. Who baked the cookies? Was it the person who decided to bake them and did the shopping? Was it the person who measured and mixed the ingredients? Was it the one who put the dough on the cookie sheet? How about the person who noticed that they were burning? Or the one who finally tasted them and decided to share them? Everyone had a hand, so at the end of the day everyone can say that she baked. Participating in an activity can be as complex or as simple as a person's abilities allow. Even a person who raises her feet to let you past with the vacuum cleaner is involved in house cleaning, that is if we are conscious of it and draw attention to her involvement. A person who is no longer able to perform a complex task can still hold an instrument, pass something, or just watch an activity in progress. All the while she is involved, and can hear the words "would you please" and "thank you" directed to her.

Involving a person in things is also a way that a caregiver can get a much needed chore done, while still keeping track of a loved one who wants to be active and helpful. One gentleman kept his wife involved while he worked on the car by asking her to please hold a tool for him. Any way she held it was just fine, so she could not fail. When she became tired of holding it, he asked her to hand it to him, thanked her, and passed her another one with the request to hold onto that one for him. All the while, they kept up a conversation or listened to music on the car stereo. He got the car maintenance done and she was happily engaged and feeling useful. Another caregiver was able to keep her husband with her while grocery shopping by asking him to please push the cart because the arthritis in her shoulder made it hard for her to do. He would not normally have volunteered to push a shopping cart. He would not have considered it appropriate for him to be doing a "woman's job," but the fact that his wife needed his help made it acceptable for him, and she in turn was pleased to have him close by.

Realize That the Objective Has Changed and Failure-Proof the Task

The paramount consideration in any activity that we do with or offer to a person who has Alzheimer's disease must be the quality of his experience while he is doing it. Therefore, we aim as much as possible to help the person avoid failure. In fact, whether the person experiences success or failure at a task depends almost entirely on the way we set things up. We can influence the situation in a number of ways.

We must anticipate and eliminate possible chances for error, because we cannot rely on the person to make accurate decisions and recognize errors in time. Therefore, remove any equipment or materials that can be misused, and leave only the appropriate items within sight or reach of the person. If Granny is going to polish the silver, make sure that she cannot accidentally use steel wool instead of the silver buffer.

We must also examine our standards and preconceptions about how things should be done. If we are concerned that the job be done a certain way, we should make sure that the person shares our standards and is capable of meeting them. If there is any doubt, we should consider relaxing our standards. Otherwise, we may be setting the person up for failure, and ourselves for disappointment or worse. The person's lack of judgment, poor attention, and inability to stop and start an activity appropriately will interfere with her ability to do the job as she used to and can lead to unfortunate outcomes for the caregiver who is unprepared. For example, before you ask her to trim a bush, make sure that she remembers how it is to be trimmed. Or, if you feel that she would really enjoy the task, let her do it only if you don't really mind how this particular bush is trimmed, even right down to the ground. The disastrous outcome in this case would not only be the loss of an ornamental bush, but also the person's sense of failure and uselessness, and the caregiver's frustration and sadness. Most disastrous of all, though, would be the potential rift that the episode could create between two people who are very important to each other.

There are several ways to approach this issue. Many caregivers report a gradual change in their standards. They find that it ceases being important to them to have things done a certain way. Some even find relief and pleasure in the freedom that they discover in letting go. Another way of accommodating is to take a flexible view of success, to see success where before we might have seen failure. Here is an example: Granny and the kids had been watching a watermelon ripen in their garden all summer. Finally, they went to harvest it, but wondered how they would tell whether it was ripe. This was the first time they had grown a watermelon, so none of them really knew. In her eagerness to get the melon, little Jenny dropped it and juice and red pulp splashed onto the gravel path. "It's ripe!" exclaimed Granny. "Well, now we know how to tell!" added Joey. Instead of failing to deliver a watermelon, they had succeeded in finding out whether it was ripe. Life abounds with examples of people who have snatched victory from the jaws of defeat. People coping with Alzheimer's disease must do a lot of that to stay on an even keel.

Another way to avoid defeat is to choose activities that are failure-proof. One caregiver wanted to remove a hedge from the garden. She saw an opportunity for her husband to enjoy himself in a failure-proof job. He loved the activity of trimming, but lacked the judgment to do it independently. Now that the hedge was to go, he could trim to his heart's content. After several weeks of clipping and bagging, the eyesore was gone. When the garden service people came to remove the stumps, there was little left for them to do. Other failure-proof activities are raking leaves, mopping, dusting, polishing silver, and washing and drying dishes. There is very little that can go wrong with these tasks. Other failure-proof activities can be set up. A digging plot in the garden, for example, never gets seeded but is turned over regularly by a gentleman who loves to garden but can no longer take on the full responsibility. His wife gives him compost material from the kitchen to dig into it every day.

Caregivers are often fearful of letting a cognitively impaired person handle objects that might be broken, such as china or glassware. Plastic replaces porcelain and crystal. The person is left to dry only the pots and pans, and deprived of the pleasure of handling the precious things that could make dish drying really pleasurable. Sometimes these restrictions are reasonable, if the person's motor coordination is impaired, or if her

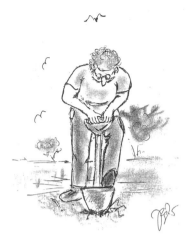

You can't really make a mistake digging up a garden plot.

judgment is so faulty that she may mishandle the items. Too often, however, these restrictions are imposed prematurely, out of anticipatory fear by the caregiver. In our Tea Group (Chapter 12), we were warned that the ladies would break the china. They never did. Their hands remembered how to handle china and they did it well. Of course, there is always the danger that a cup or glass might fall and break. This could happen to anyone and it does happen to cognitively impaired persons, but not because they are cognitively impaired.

Whenever we create "make-work" jobs for a loved one, it must be done with caution. Such activities are appropriate only when the person can still appreciate the joy of doing but is no longer concerned with the outcome. Otherwise we run the risk of affronting the person by asking them to do a meaningless chore. Even though most caregivers have good judgment when it comes to evaluating the ability of their loved one to make this distinction, many still feel guilty and question if they have not overstepped the bounds of respect. For example, one gentleman had had a difficult day and looked forward to his time with the paper while his wife did her customary chore of washing the dishes. Either the paper was particularly interesting, or she washed the dishes particularly quickly that day, but he needed a few more minutes. So, he took the already clean dishes, handed them back to her, and said, "Here, honey, here are some more." She took them and happily rewashed them, and he went back to his paper, feeling guilty, but enjoying the extra bit of rest. When he discussed this with his counselor, he realized that he had made the request of his wife based on a good understanding of her level of insight. Had he had any suspicion that she would know that the dishes had already been washed, he would not have asked. Had she called him on it, he would have apologized for his absent-mindedness and would have just helped her put them away.

Taking Risks

One of the most taxing aspects of caring for a person with Alzheimer's disease is the extraordinary amount of vigilance needed. Although we take every possible precaution to avoid failure, there are very few tasks that are totally failure-proof. At some point, all caregivers must decide how much risk they are willing to take to preserve their loved one's sense of independence and efficacy. One must also decide how much cleaning up or repairs one wants to do. It was this kind of thinking that led one gentleman to set aside a room for his wife to do her sewing. She removed buttons from some garments, sewed them back onto others, sorted, folded, snipped, and stitched for hours each day. He was willing to tidy the room every once in a while, but otherwise let her have free rein. Whatever was damaged, he felt was worth the pleasure she derived and the few hours of freedom from worry that it gave him.

Another decision a caregiver must often make is how much to risk the cognitively impaired person's safety for the freedom to continue doing things. Such a decision was made by a gentleman who let his wife continue ironing. She had never burned anything or misused the iron. He knew that some day she might, but in the meantime, he bought her an iron with an automatic shutoff and let her continue with one of her favorite jobs.

When to Just Let Her Be

There is much to be said for quiet contemplation, sitting and thinking. If a person is content, comfortable, and serene just sitting quietly, why disturb her? Why impose our standards of what is time well spent? Everyone needs private time to just be with one's own thoughts. It is not uncommon for older persons to spend more time in contemplation, sizing up their lives and achievements. This is, after all, one of the tasks of old age.

This quiet sitting or strolling is very different from the undirected wandering and restlessness we see in a person who feels the need to do something, but cannot identify an interest or find a focus for her energy. This is the distinction on the basis of which we should decide whether to offer an activity or not. Left on her own, a restless, wandering person may become agitated or get into something that leads to trouble and an experience of failure. By the same token, the person whose time is over-programmed can become overwhelmed, resentful, and resistant. The objective is to find a happy balance and avoid the distress caused by either extreme.

Evaluate the Person's Ability to Plan and to Cope with Options

"So what do you want to do today?" is probably one of the hardest questions for anyone to answer day in and day out. It is especially diffi-cult for someone who is unable to deal with abstract ideas and has poor memory and judgment. This person will usually respond with a habitual phrase, suggesting some activity from the past which may no longer be appropriate or within her abilities. This reliance on the cognitively im-paired person to identify activities also limits the scope of options to the familiar and the habitual. If the person is frequently asking to do things that exhaust her or her caregiver, or if her choices seem to be very lim-ited, the caregiver should consider taking the initiative and offering ac-tivities. This still leaves the person with the option to either accept or decline. This kind of initiative is frequently difficult for a caregiver who has been accustomed to the less dominant role in the leadership. Look-ing to the person with Alzheimer's disease to set the agenda for the day, even if it is no longer appropriate, is often the continuation of a lifelong pattern for the wife who is used to deferring to her husband's decisions or for the family housekeeper who has now become a care provider. It can be a very hard pattern to alter, since it requires a conscious and often difficult role shift for the caregiver.

Set Up a Routine and a Comfortable Rhythm

The issue of over- or underprogramming, as well as that of setting an appropriate and comfortable agenda for the day, can be dealt with by establishing a routine. Our lives feel comfortable when there is a rhythm, when one thing leads to another in a familiar way. There are times, of course, when we might feel that we are "in a rut" and have the urge to try something new and different. But for a person with cognitive impairment, a comfortable routine is a tremendous source of security. The word "comfortable," of course, is important here. When things flow predictably from one activity to another, the person can relax. Her body seems to anticipate the next event without apprehension or distress. The need to cope with the unknown, which is a real stressor, disappears. We see this comfort with routine in young children, too. We also see their distress when the routine is broken. Routine gives a person the confidence of knowing what comes next. It offers a sense of control, and it is also one of the strongest orientation devices. When a person is no longer able to tell time, she knows that after lunch it is time to go get the mail, for example. She knows that when the schoolkids get off the bus in front of the house, tea will be ready soon and she'll have a snack with her housekeeper. These kinds of routines and rhythms automatically insinuate themselves into each of our lives. The point here is to recognize their value to a person with Alzheimer's disease, and support their presence in that person's life.

The Activity Must Be Meaningful

When we are at the point of choosing an activity, we realize that not all activities are equally appealing to everyone. If we are to enjoy doing something we must find it meaningful. But how can we determine how meaningful an activity is likely to be to someone else? When having to identify enjoyable activities for someone whose ability to choose or state preferences is limited, a caregiver may find that, despite their intuition and knowledge of the person, it is helpful to have some objective criteria. These criteria are not presented in order to limit or prejudge any choice, but to serve as guidelines for selecting and evaluating an activity. In order to be meaningful, an activity must be voluntary, purposeful, socially appropriate, successful, and pleasurable. How an activity meets these criteria, of course, depends on the person doing it and the way it is done. Let's look at each of these criteria individually.

First, the activity must be voluntary. One seldom finds satisfaction in an activity that has been forced or that is done under duress. There is, however, a difference between resistance that is the result of not knowing what is being asked, or fear of getting involved in something that one will not be able to do, and an honest, informed refusal to participate. In a subsequent section we will discuss, in more detail, techniques for overcoming the recalcitrance that can be so much a hallmark of Alzheimer's disease. However, a person should not be pushed to participate in an activity to which she really objects.

Second, there must be a purpose to the activity which is obvious to the person involved and of which that person approves. There are activities that we do just because they feel good and are fun in themselves. However, being asked to do something to which we see no point is dissatisfying and demeaning. There are times when the task might have an obvious objective, but due to poor memory, insight, and analytical skills, a person with Alzheimer's disease fails to perceive it, and so finds little satisfaction in doing the activity. It is important that whoever is helping the person in the task be sensitive to her perception of the purpose. A homemaker was helping one lady to make Jell-O for dessert. As she coached her through one step to another, it was obvious that the lady had no idea what she was doing and why. As far as she was concerned, stirring colored powder into hot and cold water was something one would ask a child to do. She was going to have no part of this foolishness, and let her helper know this in no uncertain terms.

Third, a person must perceive a task as being appropriate to her social image of herself. A man of the old school, for example, may object to being asked to do something which he perceives as "woman's work." A person who is desperately trying to hold on to her sense of competence and yet feels it relentlessly slipping away, may be distressed at being asked to do something that seems childish to her. During one craft session, the group leader put some markers out on the table. Without realizing it, she had brought markers with the Crayola trademark. To one lady, this was synonymous with kindergarten. She became very affronted and left the room in a rage. A person's response depends very much on her values and sensitivities. Being asked to do a child's puzzle may not bother one person, whereas it may be a grave insult to another.

Even if a person is no longer sensitive to this aspect of an activity, there is the issue of what kind of image she projects to others while engaged in the task. Is it important to preserve the person's dignity when she is no longer aware that it is in jeopardy? This is a question that all caregivers must answer for themselves. It is sometimes difficult to find activities that are within the abilities of a very disabled person and yet are not reminiscent of children's playthings. One family who saw that their grandfather enjoyed putting together pieces of a children's plastic construction set, but were unhappy to see him lose his dignity, gave him a bag of black PVC piping. It gave him just as much enjoyment but was more appropriate for their granddad.

Last, the activity must be intrinsically pleasurable. Whereas a healthy person can anticipate a good outcome from an activity that is in itself painful or unpleasant, a person with memory loss experiences only the here and now. There is no future gain for present pain in this person's experience.

Take Clues from the Past

Old interests and hobbies are a clue to what a person may enjoy doing. Care must be taken, though, not to confront the person openly with lost skills and failing abilities. Producing a doily filled with errors may be devastating to a woman who used to pride herself on her crochet skill. One former photographer dissolved into despair upon discovering that he could no longer figure out how his prized Hazelblatt camera worked. The homemaker who had thought that he might enjoy reminiscing about old times was taken aback and could only console him. Remember that a person's personal standards measure success or failure, and an old-time favorite activity may no longer be appropriate.

By the same token, do not exclude an idea because a person never liked it in the past. People with Alzheimer's disease are no more static in their interests and tastes than anyone else. In fact, the loss of inhibitions and capacity to make judgments sometimes overrides old standards.

Whereas old, complex skills may be lost, the ability to perform simple, repetitive tasks that are familiar and, in a sense, overlearned, usually remains. These can be a treasure of activities for a family care provider, visiting homemaker, or day program staff. Most women who have raised families can fold laundry, roll pastry, or knead dough with little difficulty despite even significant cognitive impairment. Playing the piano, operating an adding machine, and shuffling and dealing cards are other examples of abilities that usually remain. There are also other, often overlooked, abilities that can be exploited. Holding an opinion and offering advice are things that most people can continue doing for a long time. We need not take the advice but we can still give a person the pleasure of giving it. The ability to experience emotions, both pleasurable and otherwise, is usually still present. Even when a person has become very impaired, the appreciation of sensory stimulation remains. A person who can no longer make out spoken or written words is usually still able to enjoy music and pictures. These can be presented as simply and in as focused a fashion as the person requires. For example, when a person becomes too distracted to listen to the radio, a tape of favorite music played on a cassette with headphones will enable her to continue to enjoy music. When magazines become too complex, a simple picture book dedicated to a favorite and familiar topic, such as flowers, dogs, or planes, can still be enjoyed. Smell, taste, and touch are senses that require little interpretation, and so remain as a source of much potential pleasure well into a person's illness.

Overcoming Resistance or Inertia

Resistance to being involved or participating in activities is one of the most frequently voiced frustrations among both family and professional caregivers. This resistance can come from a number of sources. A person with cognitive impairment may not understand what is being asked. She may not understand the words, or may not be able to conceive what to do or how to do it in the absence of any concrete physical cues. Resistance to being involved can also come from fear of the unknown. If you have no idea what the consequences of your doing something might be, you are apt to decline an invitation. The inability to organize complex motor acts, called apraxia, is another source of apparent resistance. A person who is apraxic cannot organize her body to perform an action. She relies on some outside cue to get the pattern of movement started.

Sometimes the simple act of asking a person to do something confronts her with a difficult task. Deciding whether to participate can in itself be a daunting task for a person whose information processing skills are impaired. In the Tea Group program, we found that when the ladies were asked whether they wanted to come to tea, they would usually decline. However, if they were told that tea was being served and that their company would be much appreciated, they usually accepted the invitation.

We might also inadvertently be asking a person with deceptively good social skills to perform a task that is really beyond her abilities. Finally, we might be offering her something that she does not want to do.

From this insight into the factors that may cause a person to decline an invitation, we can develop some strategies. Don't ask the person; direct and inform. She still has the option to say no. Give strong, concrete cues. This helps the person better understand what is being asked. Initiate the activity with the patient watching; this provides even stronger visual cues. It also lets her figure out whether the activity will appeal to her and gives her some specific ideas about how it is done. Trigger an automatic reaction: hand a person a spoon to start them eating, hold out a coat to trigger the act of putting it on. Finally, be sure that the activity is within the patient's ability to understand and perform. Having covered all these possibilities, if we still encounter resistance it is likely that the person really does not want to participate in the activity.

So What to Do?

All this having been said, what do we do? The following is just a sample of the sources from which potentially enjoyable activities can be gleaned.

Chores, indoors and out, are often simple repetitive tasks with which a person is very familiar. Whereas they may once have been a burden, they can now be a source of gratification, an opportunity to contribute, or a way to get some exercise. They are often, if we temper our standards, failure-proof activities. Mopping, dusting, raking leaves, polishing furniture, and taking out garbage are among the many household jobs that cannot really be done wrong.

Work simulation is a way of using old skills and interests to occupy a person who is no longer able to take on the whole job. We have already

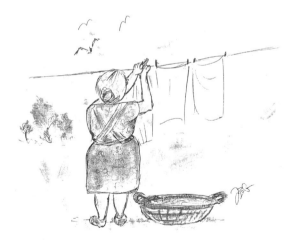

Even though they have a dryer, Harry encourages his wife to hang out the wash. She now enjoys getting out to do a job that used to be a chore.

mentioned the digging plot. Another gentleman, who had run an auto garage, spent several hours each day perusing a parts catalogue and marking off his order. He also enjoyed straightening nails. A lady enjoyed going through papers and files that were kept at a desk for her. Sorting buttons, nails, or nuts and bolts of various sizes, or pairing socks can be other such activities.

Games can still be fun if you put aside the rules and use them as a time to be together. Simplified card games such as War can still work quite well.

There must also be time for quiet activities, such as listening to music or watching films. We choose films over TV because it is more likely that a person will be able to follow and enjoy old familiar movies. Another consideration is the frequency with which persons with Alzheimer's disease confuse the events on TV with real life. In the old days, after all, TV was little and in black and white. Now with big screens and color, the action looks very lifelike. It is distressing when a person comes to believe that the crimes and disasters that take up so much airtime are actually occurring in her living room.

Intergenerational activities give a person the opportunity to enjoy children's games, songs, and silliness, yet still preserve her adult demeanor. Is that not why many of us like to take children tobogganing or to see Walt Disney movies? Everyone enjoys shedding adult decorum and being a kid again. The company of children makes this easy.

Volunteer work is a way to be useful. Many volunteer jobs, such as stuffing envelopes, opening mail, and folding newsletters, are within a cognitively impaired person's abilities. She may need to be accompanied at the task, but participation in charities and benevolent organizations is a way of staying in touch with the community and earning the gratitude of others.

Worship usually remains an important source of comfort and joy despite even severe mental impairment. Unfortunately, it is often a person's inability to stay for the entire service or follow the celebration that puts an end to her participating. Any way that the person can be accommodated to continue should be encouraged.

Reminiscence was at one time discouraged as a way of living in the past. Now we understand the importance of reviewing one's life, coming to terms with its successes and failures, and making peace. Especially at a time when the events of the present day may make little sense, recalling the joys, accomplishments, and adventures of the past can do much to support a person's sense of self. Reminiscence is also a way of passing

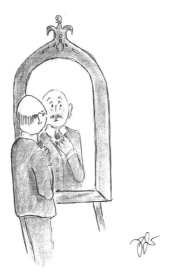

Now *that* is a good-looking guy!

one's oral history down to the next generation, a practice that used to be much respected and cherished.

Most of us are inclined to rush through the processes of showering and shaving or applying makeup. Seldom do we take the time to pamper ourselves and really enjoy these daily activities. If it is presented in a pleasurable way, however, taking care of the body is one of the basic sensory experiences that a person with Alzheimer's disease can still enjoy.

Share the Load

A final word to the caregiver at home is, "Share the load." Get someone else in or get the person you are caring for out. Ask other family members to help. Find a volunteer, either local kids or community volunteers. If possible, hire help. Get together with other caregivers and either share the costs of a sitter or let your loved ones visit.

15 | Visiting Well

Visiting grandparents, parents, friends, and other loved ones under normal, healthy circumstances is usually a treat. It keeps families and friends in touch. It lets grandparents enjoy their grandchildren, and it gives the grandchildren another set of adults who love them and even spoil them a little. Visiting a loved one in a nursing home should be a continuation of the caring relationship. It should never be a burden or a duty. Similarly, a visit from loved ones should be something to look forward to and never an upsetting event. Unfortunately, visits to a long-term care facility, particularly when a person has cognitive impairment, are often less than wonderful for everyone concerned.

One of the major sources of tension is the fact that there is usually little to talk about during a nursing home visit and even less to do. It is difficult to relate to a person who has changed so much. She might not always recognize the visitors or the people they are talking about. Removed from her customary surroundings, perhaps not even wearing her usual wardrobe, she may seem to have lost her identity. Conversation stalls, comes to a dead end or, even worse, becomes mired in complaints. Visitors may find themselves thinking of the old days, comparing the person to the way she used to be, and mourning the loss. They look around and see things that are not quite the way they want them for her, and start wondering about the quality of her care. They stay as long as they can, and then go off hoping that the next visit will be better and listing the concerns that they want to talk to the staff about the next time they come.

In this chapter we look at things that visitors can do and talk about while visiting, so that the visit is a little more like the get-togethers or trips to Granny's that everyone remembers and used to enjoy. These ideas aim to help families and friends make the most of visits for both themselves and for the person they are visiting. They are also offered to facility staff and administrators, so that they can advise families and work with them to institute some of the practices and programs that can make visiting more comfortable all around. Good care is contingent, after all, on the facility staff and family members being able to work together and complement one another's roles.

Plan the Visit

It is usually the host who sets the pace of a visit, welcomes the guests, and plays the lead role. In a nursing home visit, the "host" has few resources. When there is cognitive impairment, the person receiving the visit is at an even greater disadvantage. Therefore, the visitor must take the initiative and be prepared to set the pace, start and keep the conversation going, and suggest activities or refreshments—in other words, to take charge. We have mentioned frequently in other chapters, and cannot state often enough, that when taking charge we must always be careful to preserve a person's sense of control and of her role as a valued and respected person. Taking charge does not mean reducing the other person to a passive position or in any way diminishing her capacity to contribute. On the contrary, it means taking responsibility for the event and ensuring the best possible outcome for everyone.

The best possible outcome for a person being visited might be an opportunity to feel like a hostess again. What a pity to see a lady who used to fuss over her guests gradually sink into a passive role when visitors come to call. One family, distressed at seeing this happening to their mother, made a point of encouraging her to continue hosting family visits. They brought her tea service from home, left her a cache of biscuits to serve to company, and helped her to fuss as she was used to doing. Even though she needed the occasional reminder and some prompts along the way, she greatly enjoyed her old, familiar role. Her family took charge of the situation to ensure that their mother felt as though she was, once again, in charge of the situation.

Establish a Routine of Visiting

Try to visit at a regular time. This makes your visits predictable to both the staff and the person you are visiting. Predictable routine is one of the most useful orientation devices we can offer a person with cognitive impairment. It gives the day and the week a structure, and allows the person to prepare herself, perhaps not consciously, but subliminally, for the next event. Predictable visiting times also help the staff to get the person ready for the visit. Some cognitively impaired persons fret if told too far in advance of an upcoming event. Others may take a long time warming up to an event if they are not adequately prepared. When visits are predictable, staff and family members can work out the best method of alerting the person to ensure that she is in an optimum frame of mind when the visitors arrive.

Family members sometimes feel that they would like to visit at irregular intervals to get a good overall picture of their loved one's life in the facility. Indeed, they must be welcome to stop in any time. The actual visit with the person, however, should be considered separately. It is difficult to generalize, but, for the most part, unscheduled visits tend to be more upsetting than satisfying. Although some people may enjoy the reassurance of having someone just stop in to see how they are doing, most persons with cognitive impairment take a long time to orient to an unexpected event. Then, just as they have figured out what is going on, it is time for the visitors to go. This can be perplexing or upsetting, and may leave the cognitively impaired person in an unsettled state for the rest of the day. An unexpected visit could also interrupt the person in some other activity, with the consequence that she will have to choose between continuing with the activity and seeing her visitors. The choice itself can pose a tremendous burden to a person who has limited resources. Make sure that you know how the person is likely to react before dropping in on her.

A consistent routine to the visit itself will be just as helpful to the person as regular visiting times. If the visit comprises several activities that follow one another consistently, the person will eventually become familiar with the routine. A lot depends, of course, on the person's temperament and what she is accustomed to doing, but here are a few examples. If the first few minutes of a visit tend to be tense and uncomfortable, it might be a good idea to start off with a fairly concrete, familiar, and pleasurable activity such as a manicure. Going for a walk or a short outing can be another regular part of the visit. Having a cup of tea together before leaving might be a good way to prepare the person for ending the visit. Each time you visit, note the things that the person enjoyed and the things that she seemed to anticipate with pleasure. Try to identify the cues by which she anticipated them and build them into your routine of visiting.

Conversation

Our normal pattern of social interaction already creates a routine of sorts in the rituals of greeting. "Hi. How are you?" "Just fine, thank you, and you?" "Well, thanks." These are all part of the overlearned patterns that a person usually retains for a long time even in the face of severe cognitive impairment. But what is there to say once the opening rituals of conversation are over? An important part of taking charge is controlling the conversation. After all, it is the quality of the conversation that usually determines the general tone of the visit. Here are some useful guidelines that help keep things positive.

It is usually best to avoid open-ended questions, which can put a cognitively impaired person on the spot. They demand an answer from someone who may no longer be able to recall the necessary information accurately, but does not realize it. This can cause an uncomfortable situation. For example, "What did you have for lunch today?" is a question that anyone should be able to answer. The memory-impaired person, who cannot remember lunch, still feels compelled to respond, but what can she say? She can either dismiss the question and just say, "The usual," or she can try to account for the void in her memory. What could be some logical reasons why a rational person would not remember having had lunch? It could be because the meal was really bad and not worth remembering, and so she would answer, "Terrible stuff, the food here is dreadful." Or the other possibility is that she had never had lunch, and would then answer, "I have not had any lunch today." All of these answers are drawn from the person's logical thought processes, forced by an open-ended question that she could not answer accurately. None of them tells us what she had for lunch. Not only that, a negative situation has been created out of nothing.

A better approach is being prepared to tell, instead of expecting to be told. Regarding the lunch situation, for example, find out what was on the menu. Then you can still talk about the meal, but more realistically and with better information. "I see that you had fried fish for lunch today. I remember that you used to like that. Did you enjoy it today?" At least this way, the person has a prompt and may actually remember the meal.

Keep the information pertinent. Current events may mean nothing to a person who has little memory and even less physical contact with the world outside the home. When bringing the person up to date on things, keep in mind what will be relevant to her. During the Apollo 12 moon landing, Mr. Twiggy, one of our more active residents with a moderate cognitive impairment, insisted that the whole thing was a hoax and that all the people who were glued to the TV had been utterly taken in. The more staff tried to convince him of the facts, the more irate he became, until, having convinced himself that everyone had gone mad, he shut himself in his room to escape these lunatics. Perhaps less dramatic but equally important is that listening to the latest news about people you don't remember is not only boring, it can provoke tremendous anxiety if you have some inkling that you ought to know these names but do not. To avoid such anxiety, make sure the person recognizes the people and places being discussed. When you mention people by name, briefly identify them and their relationship to yourself or to the person you are visiting.

To make things even more pertinent, try to illustrate what you say with concrete examples, pictures or objects. This is where having planned the visit is helpful. Show pictures of people to flesh out family news. Bring in samples of any projects you have under way; show the person swatches of fabric, patterns, or paint chips as you describe what you are doing.

The topics of conversation that tend to be the most pertinent to a memory-impaired person concern events from the distant past. There was a time when we used to disdain talk about the old days, considering it useless living in the past. We now realize that reminiscence is a valuable process, especially for a person who can make little sense of the here and now. The past represents the wealth of her experience, the accomplishments and contributions that she can share and pass down to the next generation. It also represents the disappointments and heartaches with which she must come to terms. It is, especially, an opportunity to savor and enjoy again the memories that she spent a lifetime creating.

As much as we encourage reminiscence, we should not force recollections. It can be painful when a loved one fails to remember events in her life that may have been very important to you. One may be inclined to insist on her trying to recall. Such pressure, as well meaning as it may be, can cause the person distress. Instead of trying to share the memories, relive them with the person by telling her what you remember of those times and how it influenced you. This is another time when it is more appropriate to give information. Here again, concrete support for what you are telling about is helpful. Bring in family picture albums, with the names of people and descriptions of the events.

Conversation is by nature an exchange, and so there must also be an opportunity for the cognitively impaired person to contribute. The main reason why we try to control the conversation is to ensure that the person has that opportunity, but we also want to make sure that she experiences success and, as much as possible, is spared frustration and embarrassment. We can ask the person to tell us things and choose topics about which we know she enjoys talking. Then, of course, we must be prepared to listen. Old stories from the past, even if they are told over and over, can be a great source of pleasure for a person who has little opportunity to express herself. Her delight in telling can be a joy to the listeners as well, even if they already know the tale by heart. Being asked to give advice and opinions about things, even controversial things, gives a person another opportunity to express herself. Because an opinion can never be wrong, it is a safe topic. We need not agree with her opinion or take her advice, but in asking the person what she thinks, and by hearing her out, we tell her that she is still valued. This is a precious gift to someone who is gradually losing independence and abilities.

Sometimes, despite all our efforts, the conversation turns sour. The person seems for some reason to become irritable and may withdraw or lash out with no apparent provocation. One of the most common culprits in this situation is the "fifth wheel conversation." This happens when two or more visitors lapse into conversation among themselves, and the cognitively impaired person, who cannot keep up, becomes excluded. Even though everyone may be speaking the person's language, if she cannot follow, the effect is the same as if they were speaking in a foreign tongue. If the person is already feeling vulnerable, this can incite feelings of paranoia. She may suspect that things are going on behind her back or that people are purposely excluding her. She may put the proverbial two and two together and unhappily get five. This distress can eventually precipitate what we perceive as a totally unprovoked attack. Keeping the person involved, reflecting back to her what is going on among the other visitors, and being alert to signs of fatigue or stress are the best ways to avoid such an unfortunate occurrence. Of course, it is never appropriate to hold conversations in the person's presence that intentionally exclude her, or to assume that she does not understand what is being said. If you notice that the conversation has left the person behind and your efforts to engage her are failing, do not persist. It is usually best to back out graciously, let the person save face, and turn the conversation to something that she will be able to follow. ·

One of the most commonly reported irritants among visitors to persons with cognitive impairment is the repetition—repetitive questions and repetition of stories or complaints. What to do about it? Very little. Repetition is part and parcel of living with a memory loss. People around a memory-impaired person must learn to listen to repetitive stories, respond to repetitive questions, and repeat essential information. It is just like making the bed; you make it every day knowing that it will not stay done and that the next day you will have to make it again.

We have already touched briefly on some of the possible sources of complaints or negative feedback from a cognitively impaired person. Although the person's memory loss and misunderstanding of complex situations may contribute to her negative perception of things, many complaints and hurt feelings come from actual incidents. Sometimes the offending situation can be rectified and sometimes it cannot. Before attempting any intervention you must have the facts. Put these facts together with what you know about the person's personality, habits, former lifestyle, value system, and current cognitive abilities. Only then will you have some insight into what is probably happening and what can be done about it. Here is an example.

One gentleman complained to his daughter that one of the nurses had made inappropriate sexual advances toward him. How should she react? Should she tell her father that such allegations are preposterous? Should she complain to the nursing staff? Neither extreme reaction addresses the situation appropriately. She told her father that she could understand how such feelings on his part would be distressing, and decided to look into the matter before going any further.

She started collecting information. She recalled that her father had always been a very private person, extremely modest and reserved. In addition, he had been accustomed to being in charge, both at work and at home, as a store manager and as the head of his household. She realized that as his cognitive impairment progressed, he was losing his judgment and his behavior was becoming more impulsive. The nursing staff told her that he had been having bladder accidents lately and was resistant to having his clothes changed by nursing staff. He became particularly defensive and angry when approached by female nurses.

The staff used the information from the daughter to modify her father's nursing plan. The new plan specified that he be changed only by a male attendant who would use an especially gentle and deferential approach. With these accommodations, clothing changes started to go quite well. However, the gentleman still remembered the few incidents that had occurred before this plan was instituted, and he became distressed whenever he saw the female nurse he had suspected. His daughter knew that explaining the situation to her father would do little good. Her best course was to assure herself that the nursing staff had things well in hand, and that her father's comfort and dignity were no longer in jeopardy. Then she could comfort her father whenever he made these accusations and let him know that she understood his distress. She simply told him that there had been a misunderstanding and that it would not happen again. The accusations continued for a while and then gradually disappeared.

The important thing in this case was to avoid an altercation. Trying to convince this gentleman that no advances had been intended would never have succeeded. Arguments would only have entrenched him farther into a defensive position and strengthened his negative convictions about the situation. One can never win such an argument. A quarrel can only make matters worse. A good rule of thumb is to acknowledge the person's distress, offer the best possible neutral alternative or explanation for the situation, and then back off. Remarkably, many care providers have observed that the more often they successfully avoided arguments, the less often they eventually had to try. They notice that when the person encounters less resistance to her negative comments and accusations, she is less likely to interpret subsequent situations in negative terms. The incidence of complaints and accusations gradually diminishes.

When we try hard to adopt and maintain a supportive and conciliatory attitude toward someone, it is sometimes easy to slip into a patronizing tone. Always keep in mind that this person is an adult, with adult sensibilities. She will feel any hint of condescension that may creep into your voice. Therefore, under all circumstances avoid talking down to the person; remember that you are speaking to another adult.

This seems like a lot to think about while having a conversation, but conversation is, after all, an essential part of a relationship and, therefore, an important component of care. For more discussion of this topic, see Chapter 9 on communication.

Have Something to Do

Another important aspect of planning a visit is knowing what you are going to do. Plan activities that will please both yourself and the person you are visiting. The activity can be something that you do with the person, or it can be something that you do by yourself in the presence of the person. Things to do with the person might include games, projects such as organizing a family album, or giving a manicure or facial. Keep things within the person's abilities, but do not underestimate the number and quality of activities that even a very impaired person can enjoy. For example, if a person used to play cards, she will probably still be able to shuffle and deal. She may no longer be able to follow a complex game, but she may be able to play a simple game such as War. Each player puts down a card and the highest card takes the trick. It is possible to simplify virtually any familiar game. Checkers is another example. And if we relax the rules altogether, any game can be an opportunity to have a good time together. This is a situation in which children and persons with cognitive impairment seem to get along very well. The children do not yet know the rules and the cognitively impaired person has forgotten them. So no one worries about rules, or they just have fun making them up as they go along.

We often think that we should be interacting with the person during the whole time that we are visiting. In many cases this is neither practical nor even possible, especially when there is little to talk about or the person tires easily. Family members report many happy visits during which they enjoyed doing their needlepoint or crossword puzzles, or reading the newspaper. What they enjoyed the most was that the time was very much like many of the pleasant evenings they had spent at home before the person came to the nursing home.

The normal routine of a person's day offers a good source of possible activities around which to plan a visit. Bathing may have been a chore while the person was at home and her caregiver was on duty twenty-four hours a day. However, it can be a very pleasant way to share some intimate time once the person has moved to a nursing home. While it is true that bathing is one of the services that is part of nursing home care, it may also be one of the few pleasant activities left to share with the person. It can be made special by using her favorite bath fragrance and taking a little more time. Sharing a meal is another option. If the person needs help at the table, the visitor can be directly involved. These events may need to be arranged with the facility staff. The provision of personal care by visitors may require clearance with the administration. Some homes require that visitors order meals a day or two in advance and pay a small charge. In other facilities, these may be new ideas that will need consideration and accommodation. It could be an interesting opportunity for families and friends to collaborate with the facility staff and administration.

Outings can also be a regular part of a visit. The simplest trips, like going to a park to watch children play, to a public garden, or to a shopping mall or farmers' market are often the best. A cup of tea at a nearby tea room or coffee shop is often better than an elaborate meal in a restaurant. Whatever you plan, make sure that it does not overwhelm or over-tire the person. It is usually best to avoid crowded places. Make sure, too, that you keep the option to leave at any time. For example, a movie or theater where you are committed to stay for the entire performance might not be a good idea if the person could become restive within the first few moments. Once you have found several outings that the person consistently enjoys, stick to them. Do not feel compelled to search out new and exciting things to do.

Timing is important in terms of how long to stay and when to return to the facility. Make sure that the person will have enough energy for the trip back. All too often, recollection of a lovely outing is wiped out because the trip back was just too tiring. The person returns unhappy and everyone wonders if it was all worth it.

Staff members sometimes report that the person is agitated after an outing that seems, to the visitor, to have gone very well. They wonder whether such outings are advisable if they leave the person in an upset condition. Usually it is not so much the outing as the process of returning that is the cause of the agitation. The return to the facility is usually at the end of a visit. Time may be short. Quick good-byes are said, the person is dropped off, and the visitor leaves. Now the person is all too often left hanging, unable to reintegrate herself back into the facility's routine. She may go to her room, sit in the lobby, wait for dinner, or wander the halls. This is empty time. While outside, the person has been stimulated to a certain level of excitement. Her energy level was raised, but now, abruptly, she no longer has anywhere to direct that energy. It can be disorienting and is usually the cause of "postactivity" agitation. Returning the person to the facility is as important a part of the visit as the outing itself, and should be given as much attention. It is a good idea to leave plenty of time for a period of readjustment, during which the visitor stays with the person and helps her settle down. If possible, plan the return to coincide with some event, such as a meal, snack, or program. This will reintegrate the person into the nursing home environment and help to avoid that confusing void.

Leaving

Parting can be very difficult. At the very least, the departure of a visitor is a change and change is often difficult for a cognitively impaired person. This is where building into the routine an activity that alerts the person to your impending departure is useful. Your leaving then comes as less of a surprise. Usually, we can just acknowledge that leaving is hard, but find comfort in the fact that we'll get together again in a few days. It helps if you can leave something behind, such as a tape to listen to, a book to look at, a treat to enjoy, or even some personal article to hold for comfort until your next visit.

The hardest situation to cope with is when the person does not understand why she cannot go home too. Once again, no amount of reasoning is likely to convince her. Setting up the situation so that she is the one who has to leave and not you is perhaps the most consistently successful way of resolving this problem. Plan your departure to coincide with the beginning of an event that the person really enjoys. Since it is time for her to go to get her hair done, it will seem as though she has to leave you behind. Distraction is another method. Involve the person in an activity that does not include your participation and, once she is engaged, say good-bye and leave. Chances are that her interest in the activity will supersede her distress at your leaving.

Duplicity is always a dangerous route, but sometimes a little deception can prevent a lot of heartache. If you are going to use a device for leaving, make sure that the staff know of your plan and support it. Also make sure to get back to someone at the residence to find out how the strategy worked.

> One gentleman found that he could tell his wife that he had to go to the washroom. If he stayed away long enough, she forgot that he had been there and became involved in something else, and he could leave without upsetting her. He shared the idea with another gentleman who decided to try the same technique with his mother. Fortunately, this fellow had the foresight to call the floor from his car phone before leaving the parking lot. His mother was frantic that her son had been lost in the men's room. He came back right away with a tale of terrible gastric upset.

This gentleman's mother was not having difficulty coping with his departure because of cognitive impairment. She was actually angry that he had not brought her to live with him. Her resistance to his leaving was a reflection of her anger. His only recourse was to tell his mother, as calmly as he could, that he was sorry that she felt that way, but he just had to go. He had to learn to be comfortable with that. Sometimes, even when a person is cognitively impaired, there is no alternative but to just leave as calmly and gently as possible. Let the staff know that she will need a little extra TLC from them, and then leave. Call later and you will usually find that the upset did not last long.

Visiting a Severely Impaired Person

It can be very difficult to continue visiting a person who has become very cognitively impaired. What is there to do when a person can no longer interact, when we do not even know if she realizes that we are there? The reality is that we never know how much a very impaired person, even one who is almost totally unresponsive, perceives. Our presence can be a precious experience to such a person, and it would be dreadful to deprive her of that just because we are not getting any feedback. We must learn how to look for the feedback. Even though a person may no longer speak or even sustain eye contact, her body will still respond to pleasurable or noxious stimuli. Something that causes the person to relax, become more calm, or draw nearer is most likely pleasurable. Anything from which the person withdraws, or that causes her to tighten up or become tense or agitated is probably frightening or unpleasant. Familiarity with this subtle body language helps visitors to choose activities to do with the person. They will also get more satisfaction from their visits, knowing that they are really making a difference and getting through to the person.

It is best to choose activities that require little or no interpretation to enjoy. For instance, listening to a lecture is meaningless unless you can comprehend the speaker's words. On the other hand, listening to the soothing tones of a loved one's voice or to familiar and cherished music requires no interpretation and is a pure pleasure. Reading requires a high level of understanding, whereas looking at pictures requires less. The more simple, familiar, and straightforward the pictures are, the less interpretation is needed to enjoy them. The senses of touch, smell, and taste can either require interpretation or be purely sensual. We can try to identify what we feel, smell, or taste, or we can just enjoy the sensations. It is the latter aspect of the experience that we want to offer the person with severe cognitive impairment.

With these principles as guides, then, we can select activities. Here are a few examples.

- Listening to familiar music on a cassette player. Headphones sometimes help a person focus.
- Singing familiar songs together. Many persons with even severe

cognitive impairment remember the lyrics and can sing along with their old favorites.

- Praying or listening as you read familiar Bible verses.
- Listening as you read familiar poetry.
- Giving massages with fragrant oils. A simple hand massage with a pleasant lotion is a good start.
- Looking at picture books.
- Listening to your voice.
- Sitting and holding hands.
- Eating a favorite treat. One lady who responded to little delighted in the visits of her niece, who brought her liquor-filled chocolates each time.
- Your just being there. Never underestimate the power of your calm and attentive presence.

Keep in Touch with Other Visitors

Far too many families find that they are the only ones keeping in touch with their loved one once she has moved to a nursing facility. Visits from friends and more distant relations gradually peter out, likely due to the same factors that make family visiting stressful at times. Do not be afraid to keep in touch with the people who used to visit and let them know that the person would still enjoy seeing them.

Making the Person's Surroundings More Inviting to Visitors

People often resist visiting at a nursing facility because they have the impression of its being an impersonal and even depressing place. They may also feel a lack of things to do and talk about while visiting the person. There are some things that we can do to overcome this impression. Make the person's environment as inviting as possible. Even if you have become accustomed to it after frequent visiting, look at the room critically. Does it reflect the personality and history of the person as much as it could? Does it afford guests a comfortable place to sit? Are there elements in the room that suggest that guests are welcome? Try to arrange the room so that visitors do not have to scramble for chairs or perch on the bed. If that is not possible, see if the facility has a room where a person can receive visitors. The person herself may no longer be able to see to such amenities or even be sensitive to them. They will,

however, make a difference to a visitor and will contribute to the likelihood of their staying longer and returning. These changes will, therefore, indirectly affect the person's quality of life. Some may need to be
cleared with the facility's administration.

Unless there is some hazard to the person's health or to the health of
her coresidents, have some treat or small refreshment available in the
person's room. A can of peanut brittle or diabetic biscuits is something
that she can offer when people stop by. If she is unable to offer it herself,
see if you can put a sign nearby saying, "Please Enjoy" or "Help Yourself."
On festive occasions some of our residents had wreaths, appropriately
decorated for the season and covered with candies and treats, hanging
in their rooms along with a small pair of scissors. They invited visitors
to help themselves by snipping off a treat. A tray of small juice cans or
even a bottle of flavored mineral water with paper cups will make visitors
feel welcome.

A room filled with pictures and memorabilia is more likely to attract
visitors than a bare one. There is more to talk about in such a room. If the
room reflects the person, her tastes, her interests, and her history, visitors
are more likely to relate to her as an individual instead of one of the mass
of nursing home residents. One facility made a project of constructing
personal history boxes and displaying them at each resident's door. Each
box contained pictures and mementos illustrating highlights of that person's life. It served as an orientation cue by which a resident was helped
to recognize her own room. It also gave visitors some information about
the person and some starting points for a conversation.

A visitors' book is another addition to a person's room that suggests
that visitors are welcomed and appreciated. As people sign the book and
add their comments, they can also see who else has visited and when.
This can be a comfortable source of conversation material and a reminder to the memory-impaired person that people are thinking of her.
Can you imagine the desolation of not being able to recall a single visit?
How lonely it must be to feel that no one ever comes to call because you
cannot remember anyone having been there. An elaboration on the
visitors' book is a journal in which all visitors and staff note special
events or concerns. It serves as a communication tool when the person's
ability to report accurately is no longer reliable, and is part of the process
of getting the facts that was mentioned earlier.

Anything that will enhance the comfort of visitors in a person's
room will contribute positively to the person's quality of life. Many relationships between nursing home residents and visitors have developed

by chance. A relative of another resident happened, for some reason, to come into one person's room, found the encounter pleasant, and returned the next time he was there. Eventually, he became a regular visitor.

Visiting with Children

Many older persons and persons with cognitive impairment do not tolerate little children well. When they do get along, though, visits from young children can be an absolute delight, not only to the older person but also to her neighbors in the facility, to staff, and to other visitors. To work well, their visits need to be structured and kept within limits that are comfortable for everyone. A predictable and agreeable routine will give the children something to look forward to and will make the visit a positive event.

Preschoolers and young school-aged children can be very active, and their energy can be a challenge to contain. If possible, give them a place where they can be without getting in anyone's way, and where they can enjoy an activity that is set up for them. Little children cannot spend a long time just visiting one on one, especially if the person they are visiting cannot actively engage them for a sustained period of time. It is a pity, though, to cut a visit short just because a child is getting restless. To keep the child occupied and content, have available a few toys that he or she can enjoy at the nursing home. Offer them in the child's own special place only when you are visiting. That way the child is content and the older person can still enjoy watching and being with the little one. The older person may even enjoy joining the game or activity. The toys and activities you choose will depend on the age and preferences of the child. Some favorites are a doll house, a folding table and chairs with a box of colored papers, pencils, scissors, stickers, and glue sticks, and coloring books. Avoid electronic games or action toys that either beep or squawk, or that may excite the child beyond tolerable limits.

Older children may continue to enjoy having their activity center at the nursing home. They might also enjoy spending time in reminiscence with the older person, either recalling times they remember or hearing about events from the older person's youth.

The relationship between children and older adults can be very special. They can relate to one another with a freedom and mutual tolerance that is unhampered by judgments, preconceptions, or conventions. They can be spontaneous, creative, and mutually supportive in their own world that is unbound by rules of comportment, bedtimes, and fear of cavities or spoiled appetites. This relationship often transcends the effects of cognitive impairment. It seems to acquire an even more intense quality when the older person has a cognitive impairment. It could be that the person is particularly sensitive to and appreciative of the child's unconditional acceptance and lack of prejudice, and feels more free to be herself. It could be that the cognitively impaired person affects the child in the same way. However this kind of relationship develops, it is a precious gift to everyone concerned. When the person's cognitive impairment is such that this kind of relationship is no longer possible, there may still be much to be gained from bringing children to visit. We never know what or how much a very withdrawn or nonresponsive person realizes or appreciates. There could still be an awareness, at a certain level, which we cannot perceive, but which would enable the person to enjoy a child's visit. It will take preparation and someone to explain to the child what has happened to Gramma and why she behaves the way she does. The lesson of respect and compassion that this experience can teach is invaluable.

Keep in Touch with the Staff and Administration

This chapter began with a statement that good care is contingent on the facility staff and family members being able to work together and complement one another's roles. Therefore, make it a regular part of your visit to meet with staff. They have become a part of your loved one's extended family, so it is important that you know, trust, and respect one another. That kind of relationship depends on frequent encounters and good communication.

An important aspect of ongoing communication between the staff and the cognitively impaired person's family is helping the staff really get to know the person. Social histories and interest inventories that are done upon admission are painfully inadequate. Most of the information is collected at a time when everyone is stressed, so that whatever information is gathered may be inaccurate and incomplete. Without knowing the person's history, accomplishments, fears, interests, preferences, and prejudices, the staff cannot hope to give good care. This kind of information must be given slowly, bit by bit, and at times when the staff can assimilate and apply it. It comes from regular and candid conversations.

You will also find that staff can be very helpful in solving problems related to your visits. Leaving, as we mentioned, can be a problem. The staff, who have had experience with many such situations, can probably offer suggestions and help you test and refine strategies.

An open and comfortable avenue of communication will be especially important if you have to bring up concerns about your loved one's care or inquire about sensitive issues, such as was true with the example of the daughter and her father mentioned earlier. Many issues can be satisfactorily resolved if they are discussed early and candidly. Otherwise, misconceptions and prejudices creep in, relations between staff and relatives become polarized, and the person in care ultimately suffers.

No one will deny that the onus of informing families about changes in programs or care plans lies with the facility staff. Even ideal systems do, however, break down. Do not be afraid to ask why things are being done a certain way before drawing conclusions. One lady had been having difficulty coping with the morning routine of getting up and dressed to have breakfast in the dining room. The staff decided to let her remain in her dressing gown and have breakfast on the unit. Then they would have the time to let her dress more independently. It worked very well, but meant that she was often not dressed before eleven o'clock in the morning. She did not mind, nor did the staff. Unfortunately, no one had informed the family of this new program. The first time that they came in and saw her not dressed, they thought it was just an oversight. The second time, they wondered about the quality of care. The third time, they were convinced that the staff were not doing their job. This unfortunate conclusion was a consequence of poor communication.

Keep in touch with administration, too. There will be times when you might suggest changes to programs or practices, express concerns, or inquire about policies such as those we have covered in this chapter. It will be much easier to do this if you have already established a good relationship with the administrator.

More and more nursing facility and retirement home administrators are realizing that families, after having had to place a loved one, need support and help in dealing with many issues related to the placement. Many have instituted family support groups to bring families together with one another and with the staff. These groups meet regularly for discussion of the most common problems, for mutual support, and to sponsor special educational programs. If the facility with which you are associated does not have such a program, you might consider getting together with the staff and other visitors to set one up.

This kind of involvement can help lessen the anxiety that is caused by the process of placing a loved one. It can also be very demanding and draining. Therefore, make sure to keep things at a level that is comfortable and suits your lifestyle. No one should feel compelled to visit or to set up and attend groups if it causes stress. This brings us to the next issue.

Deciding Not to Visit

There are times when it is not a good idea to visit. Usually it is when you know that you really do not want to be there. We wear our feelings on our sleeves. They are often transparent to a cognitively impaired person, maybe even more so than with other people. Perhaps because the person has ceased to rely on spoken communication, she may now be more sensitive to affect and body language, and is no longer as easily fooled as someone who hears you say that things are just fine. Or perhaps it is that she has forgotten how to play the game of trying to hide feelings and letting other people think they have succeeded in hiding theirs. Whatever the reason, the person is very likely to feel that you are there under duress, and the visit will probably not go well.

If you are not feeling well, but still plan to see the person, be prepared to share your troubles. This does not mean laying out all the details of what is disturbing you, but, when asked, simply acknowledging that there is something wrong. For one thing, it is much easier than trying to hide it. For another, it gives the person the opportunity to offer sympathy or express concern. These are opportunities that come very seldom to persons in long-term care. You might be surprised at the positive effect that such an exchange has on both of you. As we have mentioned before, this is not to say that you must take whatever advice the person gives you. You can simply accept the expression of concern with which it was offered.

Taking Care of Your Own Feelings

There are many difficult feelings associated with having decided to place someone in a nursing facility. These feelings can persist for a long time and continue to make visits uncomfortable. It may be helpful to identify some of the most common ones.

No one can take care of your loved one exactly the way you did. You have had one approach, the staff in the nursing home may have another. One is not necessarily better than the other. The ideal is a melding of both, because each has a different perspective to offer. Your care is based on an intimate relationship and possibly a lifetime of experience with the person. It is also based on your knowledge of that person before she became ill. This gives you a certain insight into her habits, personality, and preferences. It can also affect your perception of her current abilities and behavior. No matter how much you try to avoid comparisons with the way she used to be, they insinuate themselves into every encounter. You know the standard to which she was capable of performing and the heights of achievement that she had reached. In comparison, the few things that she can do now may seem insignificant. The staff who know her only the way she is now naturally see her in a different light. They have no preconceptions with which to compare her present performance. They are also more free to try new approaches with her, and experiment with new foods, activities, or company. Some of these things may appeal to the person and surprise her relatives.

Be prepared for changes. Dementing illness alters the way a person perceives and reacts to things. It can also change a person's judgment and priorities. This, combined with the novel environment, can produce some remarkable transformations. Mrs. T. was a very refined lady who had never liked television. One Saturday morning her family was astonished to find her enthralled by the cartoons on TV and enjoying popcorn with a group of children who had come to visit. From then on, "Loony Toons" became a part of her family's regular routine whenever Mrs. T. went home to visit for the weekend, something that no one would ever have thought of. Another family had always considered their father a shy, retiring person, until they came in after Happy Hour and saw him clearing up ashtrays, collecting glasses, and joshing with the stragglers as though he were actually running a pub.

Also be prepared to share your loved one's affection and allegiance with others. This could be a situation in which sharing means you actually end up with more. Instead of losing a loved one to placement, many people find that they gain friends, and that their family actually grows.

16	Some Lessons That Come
	from Caring

Many lessons come our way through the experience of caring. Usually, however, the caregiver is so tied up in the day-to-day demands of the job that there is little time to reflect on and really become mindful of these lessons. Every once in a while, a little time to think on one's own can be most valuable. Caregivers have identified some lessons.

Things change. The only thing in this life that you can really count on is that things will change. Nothing lasts. No matter how hard you try to hold onto the moment that you are savoring, it eventually does slip away. So do the trials, however. Negative events are not a never-ending pattern.

If you try to hold on hard enough to the way things used to be, you stand a good chance of not seeing the good that has come out of the change that you've been resisting. "He never admitted that he needed me," said one woman. "Now that he's not always fighting for his way, I see a side of him that is new to me and I like it, despite the tragedy that has befallen us."

You are not a fortune teller. You cannot predict how anything will turn out. You may use your best judgment, and try to apply lessons learned from other situations, but you can never be sure. So don't deny yourself any possibility just because you are afraid that things will not work. Especially don't try to apply "rules" blindly. You might miss something wonderful. One lady's family was going to forgo taking their grandmother to the circus because people with Alzheimer's disease are not supposed to tolerate crowds. But in the end they did take her, and everyone had a wonderful time. Be prepared for anything, but don't count on anything either.

You are not a mind reader. You have no way of knowing what is on people's minds unless you give them a chance to tell you. We often assume what others are thinking and spend a lot of energy trying to make sure that they don't get the wrong impression. We attribute motivations to others based on our own feelings and expectations. We do this

246

with a person who has Alzheimer's disease just as much as we do it with neighbors and family. One lady resigned from her bridge group because she felt embarrassed by what she thought the others were thinking of her husband's peculiar behavior. They thought she had resigned because she didn't like them.

You are not a magician. You cannot be everything, do everything, and fix everything. If you could, you would have absolute control over everything; and if you had absolute control, you would have absolute responsibility. No one can handle such a burden. So many caregivers think that they are responsible for everything, and when they fail to deliver they feel guilty. Guilt is the biggest and most useless energy drain of all.

No matter how much you try, there are some things that you will never be able to control. Other people and their behavior is one. We can influence their behavior by our actions, but we cannot control it. Therefore, it is best to accept people as they are.

There are things that you and only you can control. One is how you feel. No one can make you feel bad, guilty, ashamed, or even good. The key is to identify the things you can control so that you can put your effort where it will bear some fruit.

The world is filled with kind people who would love to help if they only knew what you needed. No one can possibly know what you are going through. No one's imagination is good enough. Everyone wants to believe that you are coping just fine. So you have to let people know that you could use help, and tell them specifically what kind of help you need.

There is no such thing as reciprocity, especially from a person with dementia. You should not give with the expectation of getting in return. Do it for yourself, and only if you really want to. Remember, you do have control over your own feelings.

Don't judge and don't worry about being judged. Because we really don't know their true circumstances, we should not judge other people. One lady told us of having seen a man in dirty clothes and a ragged little boy walk into a liquor store with twelve cases of empty beer bottles. People in the store looked askance at the man. "Drinking like that and he can't even buy decent clothes for the boy," they muttered. She wondered which of them could have been sure that he hadn't, in fact, been up since dawn collecting the bottles from the roadside so he could buy clothes for the boy. Then she realized that just as she was unable to judge that man, no one was able to judge her and the job she was doing taking care of her husband.

No one can really know our circumstances, especially when the cognitively impaired person has such a good social facade. They cannot accurately judge us either. One caregiver said, "If I must justify myself to people, they are not worth the effort."

Every question has a thousand right answers. You just have to open your mind to the possibilities. This is even more the case with a person who has Alzheimer's disease. Freed of social constraints, she can see so many more possibilities. Where is the best place to sleep? Wherever you are comfortable when you get tired, such as in front of the TV. Do you find yourself saying more and more often, "Why not?" or "So what?" That's a good sign, because it means you are redirecting your energy and your values so that they will do the most good.

Little things mean a lot, sometimes more than the big things. For one thing, the little things happen so much more often and are so much more accessible. Life is made up of little things like getting mail, eating ice cream, and having coffee at the kitchen table. Every moment is precious, because it will never come back. Concentrate on what you are doing at the moment. If you lose the moment, you lose everything, because for the person with dementia, that's all there is.

The little things are there for us to milk and extract beauty, healing, and strength from. When a person cannot see these little things for what they are worth, that is when burnout is setting in.

Relationships mean everything. Everything is possible when there is mutual trust and respect. The person with dementia, just like anyone else, will resist control but accept guidance.

We must be prepared to change. The following quote was in a notebook one lady left with me. She had not indicated the source. "Certain coping mechanisms have been serving us for a lifetime, perhaps not well, but at least we knew how they worked. We would set our sights on an objective and move steadily toward it. There are times when we see that our objective is not where we thought it was and that is when we have to change course."

References

Âkerlund, B., and Norberg, A. 1986. Group psychotherapy with demented patients. *Geriatic Nursing* 7(2): 83–84.

American Psychiatric Association. 1994. *Diagnostic and Statistical Manual of Mental Disorders.* 4th ed. Washington, D.C.: American Psychiatric Press.

Archibald, C. 1994. *Sexuality and Dementia: A Guide.* Dementia Services Development Centre, University of Stirling, Scotland.

Arkin, S. M. 1996. Volunteers in partnership: An Alzheimer's rehabilitation program delivered by students. *American Journal of Alzheimer's Disease* 11(1): 12–22.

Barkan, B. 1981. The live oak regenerative community: Reconnecting culture within the long term care environment. *Aging* (Sept.–Oct.): 2–7.

Brody, E. M., Kleban, M. H., Lawton, M. P., and Moss, M. 1974. A longitudinal look at excess disabilities in the mentally impaired aged. *Journal of Gerontology* 29(1): 79–84.

Brody, E. M., Kleban, M. H., Lawton, M. P., and Silverman, H. A. 1971. Excess disabilities of mentally impaired aged: Impact of individualized treatment. *Gerontologist* 11(2): 124–33.

Burnside, I. 1984. Group work with the cognitively impaired. In *Working with the Elderly: Group Process and Techniques.* Belmont, Calif.: Wadsworth.

Burton, J. E. 1982. Programming to meet the needs of the elderly in institutions. *Canadian Journal of Occupational Therapy* 49(3): 89–91.

Canadian Association of Occupational Therapists. 1991. *Occupational Therapy Guidelines for Client-Centered Practice.* Toronto: CAOT Publications.

Carswell, A., Carson, L., Walop, W., and Zgola, J. 1992. A theoretical model of functional performance in persons with Alzheimer disease. *Canadian Journal of Occupational Therapy* 59(3): 132–40.

Carswell, A., Dulberg, C., Carson, L., and Zgola, J. 1995. The Functional Performance Measure for persons with Alzheimer's disease: Reliability and validity. *Canadian Journal of Occupational Therapy* 62(2): 62–69.

Case study: The forgetful mourner. 1995. *Hastings Center Report* 25(1): 32–33.

Coons, D. M., and Weaverdyck, S. E. 1986. Wesley Hall: A residential unit for persons with Alzheimer's disease and related disorders. In *Therapeutic Interventions for the Person with Dementia,* ed. E. D. Taira, 29–53. New York: Haworth Press.

Cowan, K. 1989. Care of patients with behavioural problems at the Perley Hospital: Needs assessment. Unpublished field study for M.H.A. program.

De Castillejo, I. C. 1974. *Knowing Woman: A Feminine Psychology.* New York: Harper & Row.

Edelson, J. S., and Lyons, W. H. 1985. *Institutional Care of the Mentally Impaired Elderly.* New York: Van Nostrand Reinhold.

Feil, N. 1982. *Validation: The Feil Method.* Cleveland: Edward Feil Productions.

Gilewski, J. 1986. Group therapy with cognitively impaired older adults. *Clinical Gerontologist* 5(3/4): 281–96.

Gilleard, C. J., Boyd, W. D., and Watt, G. 1982. Problems of caring for the elderly mentally infirm at home. *Archives of Gerontology and Geriatrics* 1: 151–58.

Gilleard, C. J., Gilleard, E., Gledhill, K., and Whittick, J. 1984. Caring for the elderly mentally infirm at home: A survey of the supporters. *Journal of Epidemiology and Community Health* 38: 319–25.

Gnaedinger, N. 1989. *Housing Alzheimer's Disease at Home.* Ottawa: Canada Mortgage and Housing Corporation.

Haugen, P. K. 1985. Behavior of patients with dementia. *Danish Medical Bulletin* 32 (Suppl. 1): 62–65.

Heine, C. A. 1986. Burnout among nursing home personnel. *Journal of Gerontological Nursing* 12(3): 14–18.

Hiatt, L. G. 1987. Supportive design for people with memory impairments. In *Confronting Alzheimer's Disease,* ed. A. C. Kalicki, 138–63. Owings Mills, Md.: National Health Publishing, in cooperation with the American Association of Homes for the Aging.

Keilhoffner, G. 1983. *Health through Occupation: Theory and Practice in Occupational Therapy.* Philadelphia: F. A. Davis.

Lahav, D., Vainer-Benaiah, Z., Kere, P., and Furman, T. 1996. Loss of self-personality traits in Alzheimer patients as conceived by spouses, children and the patient. Unpublished study presented at the Alzheimer's Disease 12th International Conference, Jerusalem.

Law, M., Polatajko, H., Pollock, N., McColl, M., Carswell, A., and Baptiste, S. 1994. Pilot testing of the Canadian Occupational Performance Measure: Clinical and measurement issues. *Canadian Journal of Occupational Therapy* 61(4): 191–97.

Lawton, M. P. 1984. An introduction and overview to environment. *Pride Institute Journal of Long-term Health Care* 4: 1–11.

Lerner, A. B. 1984. I've lost a kingdom: A victim's remarks on Alzheimer's disease. *Journal of the American Geriatrics Society* 32(12): 935.

Lund, D. A., Hill, R. D., Caserta, M. S., and Wright, S. D. 1995. Video Respite™: An innovative resource for family, professional caregivers, and persons with dementia. *Gerontologist* 35(5): 683–90.

Mace, N. L., and Rabins, P. V. 1981. *The 36-Hour Day: A Family Guide to Caring for Persons with Alzheimer's Disease, Related Dementing Illnesses, and Memory Loss in Later Life.* Baltimore: Johns Hopkins University Press.

Maloney, C. C., and Daily, T. 1986. An eclectic group program for nursing home residents with dementia. *Physical and Occupational Therapy in Geriatrics* 4(3): 55–80.

Opzoomer, M. A., Puxty, J., Walop, W., Teaffe, M., Fortin, C., and McLean, M.

1989. *Prevalence of Dementia in Long Term Care Facilities in Ottawa-Carleton Region.* Final Report. Ottawa: Health and Welfare Canada.

Paire, J. A., and Karney, R. J. 1984. The effectiveness of sensory stimulation for geropsychiatric inpatients. *American Journal of Occupational Therapy* 38(8): 505–9.

Peavy, G. M., Salmon, D. P., Rice, V. A., Galasko, D., Samuel, W., Taylor, K. I., Ernesto, C., Butters, N., and Thai, L. 1996. Neuropsychological assessment of severely demented elderly: The Severe Cognitive Impairment Profile. *Archives of Neurology* 53(4): 367–72.

Peck, S. 1987. *The Different Drum: Community-Making and Peace.* New York: Simon & Schuster.

Rader, J., Doan, J., and Schwab, M. 1985. How to decrease wandering, a form of agenda behavior. *Geriatric Nursing* 6(4): 196–99.

Sanford, J.R.D. 1975. Tolerance of disability in elderly dependents at home: Its significance for hospital practice. *British Medical Journal* 3: 471–73.

Sheridan, C. 1991. *Reminiscence: Uncovering a Lifetime of Memories.* Forest Knolls, Calif.: Elder Books.

Shoham, H., and Neuschatz, S. 1985. Group therapy with senile patients. *Social Work* 30(1): 69–72.

Snyder, L. H. 1978. Environmental changes for socialization. *Journal of Nursing Administration* 8(1): 44–50.

Thomas, A. 1985. Learning in society: A discussion paper. In *Learning in Society: Toward a New Paradigm.* Ottawa: UNESCO.

Woods, R. T., and Britton, P. G. 1985. *Clinical Psychology and the Elderly.* Rockville, Md.: Aspen Systems Corporation.

Zgola, J. M. 1987. *Doing Things: A Guide to Programming Activities for Persons with Alzheimer's Disease and Related Disorders.* Baltimore: Johns Hopkins University Press.

——. 1988. Therapeutic companionship: A home program for clients with Alzheimer's disease. *Canadian Journal of Occupational Therapy* 55(1): 26 30.

——. 1990. Therapeutic activity. In *Dementia Care: Patient, Family, and Community,* ed. N. Mace, 148–72. Baltimore: Johns Hopkins University Press.

Zgola, J. M., and Coulter, L. G. 1988. I can tell you about that: A therapeutic group program for cognitively impaired persons. *American Journal of Alzheimer's Care and Related Disorders and Research* 3(4): 17–22.

Index

JITKA M. ZGOLA, O.T.(C), is an occupational therapist, author, educator, and advisor to those who care for persons with Alzheimer's disease and related dementing illnesses. She has close to twenty years' experience with clients, professionals, and family care providers, in direct service and administration. She provides teaching and consultation in dementia care to agencies and professional groups throughout Canada, the United States, and Europe. She has an ongoing advisory relationship with a number of long-term care facilities and agencies that serve persons with dementia and their families. She has contributed to several publications, has written many articles, and is the author of *Doing Things: A Guide to Programming Activities for Persons with Alzheimer's Disease and Related Disorders* (also from Johns Hopkins University Press).

Library of Congress Cataloging-in-Publication Data

Zgola, Jitka M.
    Care that works : a relationship approach to persons with
dementia / Jitka M. Zgola.
        p.   cm.
    Includes bibliographical references and index.
    ISBN 0-8018-6025-3 (alk. paper). —
ISBN 0-8018-6026-1 (pbk. : alk. paper)
    1. Dementia—Patients—Care.   2. Dementia—Patients—Home
care.   3. Dementia—Patients—Services for.   4. Alzheimer's
disease—Patients—Care.   5. Alzheimer's disease—Patients—
Services for.   6. Interpersonal relations.   I. Title.
RC521.Z47   1999
362.1'9683—dc21   98-42344 CIP